Contemporary Diagnosis and Management of
Psoriasis®

Tina Bhutani, MD
Department of Dermatology
University of California Medical Center, San Francisco, CA

Judith Hong, MD
Department of Dermatology
University of California Medical Center, San Francisco, CA

John Koo, MD
Director, Psoriasis and Skin Treatment Center
Professor and Vice Chairman, Department of Dermatology
University of California Medical Center, San Francisco, CA

With Foreword by

Mark Lebwohl, MD
Sol and Clara Kest Professor and Chairman
Department of Dermatology
The Mount Sinai School of Medicine, New York, NY

Fifth Edition

Published by Handbooks in Health Care Co.,
Newtown, Pennsylvania, USA

This book has been prepared and is presented as a service to the medical community. The information provided reflects the knowledge, experience, and personal opinions of the authors Tina Bhutani, MD, Department of Dermatology, University of California Medical Center, San Franscisco, CA; Judith Hong, MD, Department of Dermatology, University of California Medical Center, San Franscisco; and John Koo, MD, Director, Psoriasis Treatment Center, and Professor and Vice Chairman, Department of Dermatology, University of California Medical Center, San Francisco; with assistance from Grace Bandow, MD; Terrence Keaney, MD; Bonnie Koo, MD; Jane Kwan, MD; Mei-Lin Pang, MD; Rupa Pugashetti, MD.

This book is not intended to replace or to be used as a substitute for the complete prescribing information prepared by each manufacturer for each drug. Because of possible variations in drug indications, in dosage information, in newly described toxicities, in drug/drug interactions, and in other items of importance, reference to such complete prescribing information is definitely recommended before any of the drugs discussed are used or prescribed.

International Standard Book Number: 978-1-935103-47-9

Library of Congress Catalog Card Number: 2010916062

Table of Contents

Foreword

D o we need yet another book on psoriasis? Anyone who reads this new edition of *Contemporary Diagnosis and Management of Psoriasis*® will answer with a resounding "yes." This handbook is replete with incredibly useful tables that concisely answer most questions that may arise when clinicians treat psoriasis.

I find myself turning to the material and tables in this book regularly. For seasoned dermatologists, there are tables listing drugs that can exacerbate psoriasis. Other tables list drugs to avoid when taking methotrexate or drugs to avoid when taking cyclosporine. When prescribing medications for patients, many of us are unaware of the sizes of the tubes our patients will receive, but these are conveniently listed in a practical table of the available sizes (in grams) of the various topical therapies we prescribe. In addition, there are tables and text that outline specific difficult situations. For example, there is a treatment algorithm for pregnant patients and a table listing treatments that are contraindicated during pregnancy. Another table proposes a regimen for treatment-resistant scalp psoriasis, a commonly encountered presentation in the office.

There are also practical guidelines and tables for the novice dermatologist and for dermatology residents, such as a list of commonly used tar preparations. Tables dealing with each of the biologic agents list the drug doses, the required laboratory tests, warnings, and precautions. This book also contains the most up-to-date ranking of commonly used topical steroids. I often consult that table even though I thought I knew the appropriate ranking for many of the topical corticosteroids that have been prescribed.

The appendix contains practice-based tables for the beginning dermatologist who is nervous about prescribing systemic agents for psoriasis. There are precise dosing and monitoring guidelines for acitretin, methotrexate, cyclosporine, biologics, and methoxsalen used in PUVA. The monitoring and dosage requirements for PUVA are likewise outlined in table form.

In summary, *Contemporary Diagnosis and Management of Psoriasis*® is one of the most user-friendly handbooks on psoriasis. It allows clinicians to quickly access critical information that they can use every day. It is well written by Dr. John Koo, a world authority on the treatment of psoriasis, and by his two associates, Dr. Tina Bhutani and Dr. Judith Hong who, though early in their careers, have already been extraordinarily productive. This book belongs on the desk of every physician taking care of patients with psoriasis.

Mark Lebwohl, MD
Sol and Clara Kest Professor and Chairman
Department of Dermatology
The Mount Sinai School of Medicine
New York, NY

Chapter 1

Introduction

P soriasis is one of the most commonly encountered conditions in dermatology practice and is regularly seen in primary care medicine. In the United States, a recent nationwide survey revealed the prevalence of psoriasis to be between 2.1% and 2.6% of the population. Psoriasis is relatively rare in childhood; patients typically develop the disease in young adulthood. Racially, psoriasis is most prevalent among Caucasians, about half as prevalent in African Americans as compared with Caucasians, and about half as prevalent among Asian Americans as compared with African Americans. Men and women are affected equally.

In most patients, psoriasis is experienced as a pruritic, inflammatory condition with a chronic remitting and relapsing course. In contrast to atopic dermatitis, which tends to improve as the patient ages, psoriasis typically remains active throughout the patient's lifetime or gradually becomes more widespread. Also, unlike atopic dermatitis, where the onset of disease is usually limited to childhood or young adulthood, psoriasis can develop at any age. First episodes of psoriasis have even been reported in centenarians.

Although a predisposition to develop psoriasis can be genetically transmitted, many cases arise in individuals with no reported family history of the disease. Several factors are known to exacerbate psoriasis, including traumatic injury to the skin, physical and psychological stress, cold weather, excessive alcohol intake, and drugs such as lithium and β-blockers. Table 1-1 provides a list of drugs that can exacerbate psoriasis.

Table 1-1: Drugs That Can Exacerbate Psoriasis

- Corticosteroids (rebound can occur upon withdrawal)
- Interferons
- Lithium (Eskalith®, Lithobid®)
- β-Blockers
- Nonsteroidal anti-inflammatory drugs (NSAIDs)
- Angiotensin-converting enzyme (ACE) inhibitors
- Antimalarials (chloroquine [Aralen®], hydroxychloroquine [Plaquenil®], quinacrine, and others)
- Gemfibrozil (Lopid®)

The pathophysiology of psoriasis involves an abnormal activation of the immune system in the skin. T cells are triggered and release cytokines, which cause inflammation of target tissues and activate more T cells, further propagating an inflammatory cascade. Many of the treatments being used or developed for psoriasis are immunomodulators, which decrease and interfere with lymphocyte activity in psoriatic skin. In addition to inflammation, the epidermis in psoriatic skin replicates up to 10 times faster than normal, and contains double the normal number of proliferating cells (which produce 30 times more cells per day than normal skin). This increased rate of cell turnover, coupled with the inflammatory process, results in the typical lesions of psoriasis.

Most patients with psoriasis suffer localized outbreaks (Figure 1-1, see color insert), especially on the elbows, knees, and scalp. However, a small but significant proportion of patients experience generalized psoriasis.

Those with localized involvement have the potential to flare, which can then lead to generalized involvement (Figure 1-2, see color insert).

Although skin disorders are often trivialized by those who do not have them, a rigorous study of the impact of psoriasis on health-related quality of life (QOL) using a validated QOL questionnaire revealed that the negative impact of psoriasis is no less than that seen in other serious, chronic medical conditions such as cancer, hypertension, diabetes, arthritis, heart disease, and depression. In fact, only congestive heart failure patients had worse physical QOL scores than psoriasis patients. In terms of impact on mental QOL, only patients with chronic lung disease and major depression scored worse than patients with psoriasis.

Consequently, it is important to learn how to manage psoriasis, not only because of its prevalence, but also because of the profound impact it can have on a patient's QOL. In addition, timely and proper intervention can prevent localized disease from becoming generalized, and, in some rare instances, reduce the risk of conversion into life-threatening erythrodermic or generalized pustular psoriasis. This book describes the diagnosis and management of psoriasis with an emphasis on optimizing treatment by using the full breadth of the therapeutic armamentarium that is now available for psoriasis patients.

Selected Readings

Menter AM, Weinstein GD: An overview of psoriasis. In: Koo JYM, Lee CS, Lebwohl MG, et al, eds. *Moderate to Severe Psoriasis*. New York, Informa Healthcare USA, 2009, pp 1-26.

Koo JYM, Kowalski JW, Lebwohl MG, et al: Evaluating psoriasis in patients. In: Koo JYM, Lee CS, Lebwohl MG, et al, eds. *Moderate to Severe Psoriasis*. New York, Informa Healthcare USA, 2009, pp 27-48.

Rapp SR, Feldman SR, Exum ML, et al: Psoriasis causes as much disability as other major medical illnesses. *J Am Acad Dermatol* 1999; 41:401-407.

Chapter 2

Diagnosing and Assessing Psoriasis

In most cases, psoriatic lesions can be diagnosed clinically without performing a skin biopsy. They are characterized by the presence of well-demarcated, scaly plaques with sharply defined borders. Psoriatic lesions are typically located on the extensor aspects of the body, such as the elbows and the knees. Other common areas of involvement include the scalp (particularly the occipital scalp) behind the ears, umbilicus, lower back, shins, nails, and the gluteal cleft. Gluteal pinking is one of the more characteristic signs of psoriasis. This is the presence of erythema ranging from pink to beefy bright red, within the buttock crease. It often lacks scales because of the moist, occluded nature of the buttock area.

An untreated psoriatic plaque consists of silvery, white, unusually thick, micaceous scales. The term micaceous is derived from the word mica, which is a mineral that crystallizes in a particular way that allows perfect cleavage into thin, silvery planes. Micaceous scales are much thicker than those found in other common scaly skin conditions such as seborrheic dermatitis (seborrhea) or atopic dermatitis (eczema). Other chronic inflammatory skin conditions such as seborrheic dermatitis, atopic dermatitis, or other forms of eczema generally lack such sharply demarcated borders. They are instead characterized by lesions with diffuse, poorly defined borders such that the examiner may have difficulty delineating the exact line between normal and diseased skin.

Nail involvement includes specific findings, such as shallow, punctate pits; oil spots; and onycholysis, which help distinguish psoriatic nail involvement from other pathologic nail conditions. These distinguishing characteristics become most important when a patient presents with nail disease only (see Chapter 12). Onycholysis is less specific for psoriasis than nail pitting and oil spots because it is often seen in other traumatic, inflammatory, or idiopathic conditions involving the nail bed.

Although psoriasis is usually an easy diagnosis based on its characteristic features, the differential is important, especially in a primary care setting where most patients present for the first time. Other diagnoses to be considered include atopic dermatitis, contact dermatitis, seborrheic dermatitis, tinea, candidiasis, pityriasis rosea, drug eruption, cutaneous T-cell lymphoma (mycosis fungoides [MF]), and pityriasis rubra pilaris (PRP).

In contrast to atopic dermatitis, which primary care physicians are likely to encounter more than any other condition in the differential, psoriasis is distinguishable not only by its morphology, as described, but also by its location. Unless psoriasis is widespread, it is typically a disease of elbows, knees, gluteal cleft, and scalp. Atopic dermatitis usually involves flexural areas such as antecubital and popliteal fossae. An atopic history, including asthma or allergic rhinitis in either the patient or family members, can also be a clue. Atopic patients often report sensitivity to environmental triggers such as dust, pets, foods, or pollen as well as a susceptibility to secondary bacterial, fungal, and viral infections. Psoriatic skin is usually not particularly sensitive to environmental elements, bacterial overgrowth, or secondary infections. Skin antigen testing will further distinguish psoriatic and atopic skin. Test results tend to demonstrate normal reactivity in psoriatic patients vs a propensity towards anergic response in atopic patients.

Psoriasis is easily distinguished from seborrheic dermatitis. Seborrheic dermatitis involves only the sebaceous, follicle-rich areas of the scalp, face (the T-zone or eyebrows and the area on and around the nose), ears, central chest, and rarely, central upper back and the groin. Seborrhea is typically poorly demarcated, pink, oily-appearing skin with yellow-brown scales. On the scalp, the scaling of seborrheic dermatitis tends to be diffuse with fine, greasy scales, commonly called dandruff, while psoriatic scalp involvement demonstrates sharply demarcated plaques typical of the lesions on the body, with much coarser and thicker scaling. On the face, seborrheic dermatitis is typically limited to sebaceous areas around the eyebrows and the nasolabial folds while facial psoriasis is less common altogether, and can be found anywhere on the face. However, clinicians should not assume that a red, scaly rash on the face of a known psoriatic patient is necessarily psoriasis. Facial seborrheic dermatitis does commonly occur in conjunction with psoriasis and is called sebopsoriasis.

Some of the more unusual skin conditions resembling psoriasis include Mycosis fungoides (MF), PRP, and a rare form of psoriasis morphologically between psoriasis and eczema called eczematoid psoriasis, or psoriasiform eczema. Mycosis fungoides is a slowly progressive form of cutaneous T-cell lymphoma that often mimics and is easily misdiagnosed as either psoriasis or eczema. The diagnosis is made by combining clinical and histologic features and often takes several years before findings become diagnostic. If suspicion is high, or if patients do not respond to treatment, repeat biopsies should be performed because they are frequently nondiagnostic during the early years of the disease. Retrospective studies have shown that a lag time from disease onset to diagnosis ranges from 4 to 10 years. Although MF occurs in any age group, it is often suspected in older patients, especially when the lesions are not as sharply demarcated or micaceous as classic psoriatic lesions.

PRP is a rare skin condition characterized by an explosive onset of highly inflammatory, erythematous, papulosquamous lesions originating on the head and descending toward the trunk and eventually the legs. This progression is different from psoriasis in which the face tends to be the last location involved. In fact, the face is spared in most psoriasis patients despite frequent scalp involvement. Patients with PRP usually have an extremely thick, smooth, waxy layer of dead skin cells on their palms and the soles of their feet, giving the appearance that their hands have been dipped in carnauba wax (Figure 2-1, see color insert). This is different from the silvery, flaky hyperkeratosis of psoriasis on the palms and soles. Patients also typically have generalized, bright salmon-colored to orange-red erythema on the trunk with characteristic small islands of spared, normal skin. Skin biopsy is helpful in differentiating PRP from psoriasis.

In rare cases, patients present with clinical manifestations consistent with both eczema and psoriasis. The plaques are not as well demarcated as psoriasis, but more demarcated than typical eczema. Scales are also morphologically between the thickness typical of psoriasis and eczema. This diagnosis of eczematoid psoriasis or psoriasiform eczema is rarely made, and patients with these features should undergo biopsies to rule out MF.

Another rare clinical manifestation of this mixed state involves hand dermatitis exhibiting both pustules suggestive of pustular psoriasis and 'tapioca' vesicles (ie, small fluid-filled bubbles) of dyshidrotic eczema (Figure 2-2, see color insert). These cases may be preferentially treated with agents that are effective for both psoriasis and eczema, such as topical steroids, ultraviolet B (UVB), or psoralen plus ultraviolet A (PUVA) phototherapy rather than treatment specific to psoriasis, such as calcipotriene (Dovonex®).

Selected Readings

Christophers E, Mroweitz U: Psoriasis. In: Fitzpatrick TB, Freedberg IM, Eisen AZ, et al, eds: *Dermatology in General Medicine*, 5th ed. New York, NY, McGraw-Hill, 1999, pp 495-533.

Epstein EH Jr, Levin DL, Croft JD Jr, et al: Mycosis fungoides. Survival, prognostic features, response to therapy and autopsy findings. *Medicine (Baltimore)* 1972;51:61-72.

Chapter 3

Types of Psoriasis

Plaque-type Psoriasis

More than 90% of patients with psoriasis have plaque-type disease. Lesions are sharply demarcated with wide-ranging degrees of erythema, induration, and scaling. When plaque-type psoriasis first erupts, lesions initially appear as tiny, well-demarcated 'islands' of scaly, inflammatory skin, which quickly coalesce to form larger plaques. While plaques can occur on almost any part of the skin (aside from the mucous membranes), they are typically found on the elbows, knees, shins, lower back, umbilicus, and intergluteal fold (Figure 1-1, see color insert). The scalp is commonly involved, especially behind the ears and in the occipital region, while the face is often spared.

Pruritus of varying severity frequently occurs but is not as consistently observed as in patients with atopic dermatitis or other forms of eczema. Some patients with widespread psoriasis experience little itching, while others with localized plaques may suffer from disruptive pruritus. Unlike the itching associated with atopic dermatitis where histamine is thought to play a major role, the pruritus of psoriasis generally does not respond well to nonsedating antihistamines such as loratadine (Alavert®, Claritin®).

Erythrodermic Psoriasis

Erythrodermic psoriasis (Figure 3-1, see color insert) involves most or all of the skin surface, manifesting as a bright erythema that causes the entire body to take on the appearance of a cooked lobster. Any patient with plaque-type psoriasis can quickly convert into erythrodermic psoriasis if he or she experiences a severe flare-up. Unlike plaque-type psoriasis, where systemic symptoms are rare, many erythrodermic psoriasis patients experience uncomfortable symptoms such as fever, chills, and rigors. Erythrodermic psoriasis can be a medical emergency, especially in the elderly. Because a large proportion of blood flow is shunted to the skin, renal failure or high-output cardiac failure is possible. Erythrodermic patients with concomitant medical conditions that are unstable should be treated in an inpatient setting.

Guttate Psoriasis

Guttate psoriasis presents as a sudden, diffuse eruption consisting of smaller, droplet-size lesions on the trunk and extremities (Figure 3-2, see color insert). It tends to occur in young adults and is often preceded by an acute bacterial infection, most commonly streptococcal pharyngitis, or by systemic corticosteroid withdrawal.

Inverse Psoriasis

The patient with inverse psoriasis experiences prominent involvement of the flexural areas, such as the antecubital and popliteal fossae, inframammary region, axillae, inguinal region, groin, and intergluteal fold (Figure 3-3, see color insert). Although these areas are often spared in the typical psoriasis patient, inverse psoriasis can coexist with regular plaque-type psoriasis. The treatment of inverse psoriasis must be carefully conducted because topical agents, such as corticosteroids, can induce atrophy, irritation, and maceration in self-occluded areas of the skin.

Pustular Psoriasis

Pustular psoriasis (Figure 3-4, see color insert) clinically manifests as psoriatic lesions that are filled with sterile pus. Because of its unique appearance, pustular psoriasis is frequently misdiagnosed as an infectious process. Patients are often kept on antibiotics for a prolonged period before the primary care physician is aware of the actual diagnosis, either through self-discovery or dermatology consultation. Pustular psoriasis is generally more difficult to treat than plaque-type psoriasis and occurs in localized and generalized forms.

Localized pustular psoriasis can be highly disabling, especially when it involves the palms and/or the soles of the feet, but is usually not life-threatening. In contrast, generalized pustular psoriasis, also known as the von Zumbusch type, is a medical emergency and should be treated accordingly. Patients with a generalized pustular flare-up can die of sepsis, renal failure, congestive heart failure, and other complications if the condition is not promptly brought under control. To prevent such sequelae, these patients should be monitored closely and if necessary hospitalized as quickly as possible with a dermatologist on consult.

Hand and Foot Psoriasis

Hand and foot psoriasis occurs as either plaque-type or pustular disease that is most severe on the palms and soles (Figures 3-5, 3-6, and 3-7, see color insert). It is challenging to manage, and patients may require phototherapy or systemic therapy in addition to topicals. The thickness of the skin on the palms and soles impairs the ability of topical medications to effectively penetrate down to the living layer of the skin. UVA rays penetrate skin much deeper than UVB rays. Therefore, hand and foot PUVA phototherapy is generally more effective than localized application of narrow-band UVB phototherapy. Although the area affected may be small, the location of the lesions makes hand and foot psoriasis disabling to the patient. As a result, more elaborate and aggressive treatment is often warranted for these patients. Besides the hands and feet, psoriasis affects other areas that require specialized treatment. Cases such as nail psoriasis and scalp psoriasis will be described in further detail in the therapy sections of this handbook.

Selected Reading

Menter AM, Weinstein GD: An overview of psoriasis. In: Koo JYM, Lee CS, Lebwohl MG, et al, eds. *Moderate to Severe Psoriasis*. New York, Informa Healthcare USA, 2009, pp 1-26.

3

Chapter **4**

Determining Disease Severity

P soriasis is classically categorized as mild, moderate, or severe. Usually, mild disease can be controlled with topical agents, while moderate-to-severe cases require the addition of phototherapy or systemic agents. One of the most important decisions that physicians need to make is whether psoriasis can be adequately treated with topical medications alone or whether it requires photo-therapy and/or systemic treatment. This key decision is made with considerations of such factors as the extent of psoriasis in terms of body surface area (BSA) involved, responsiveness or lack of response to topical agents, and the quality-of-life (QOL) impact the disease has on the patient. Another consideration is the presence or absence of psoriatic arthritis.

The palm of one's hand, including the thumb, consti-tutes approximately 1% of the total BSA. If ≥10% of the BSA is involved, it becomes tedious and time consuming to apply topical medications to all areas of involved skin. Although some patients could potentially chase after every psoriatic lesion with topical medications even if a large amount of BSA is involved, most busy, working individuals find it unfeasible to treat >10% of the BSA with topical medications alone. With >10% BSA involvement, it also becomes difficult to obtain a sufficient quantity of topical medications for adequate coverage. Moreover, frequently used topical medications for psoriasis, such as super-potent topical steroids and calcipotriene (Dovonex®), have limitations on the amount of drug that is allowed to be used per unit time for safety reasons. Ideally, any patient with ≥10% BSA involvement should be managed by a dermatologist so that phototherapy and/or systemic therapy can be made available in addition to topical treatment.

Even when the BSA involved is <10%, phototherapy or systemic therapy should be considered if the psoriatic lesions prove to be unresponsive to optimized topical therapeutic regimens. This is especially true if the localized involvement is physically disabling or emotionally, occupationally, or socially devastating to the patient. For example, a patient may have a small proportion of BSA affected by psoriasis, but if the hands or feet comprise the involved areas, the impact on QOL may be profound and aggressive intervention warranted. A person whose appearance is important to his or her occupation (such as a fashion model) may find even a single plaque of psoriasis on the face debilitating, even though the disease is not widespread.

Depending on the study cited, a range of 10% to 40% of psoriatic patients have psoriatic arthritis. A major clinical difference between psoriatic arthritis and psoriasis is that even if psoriasis is widespread, the patient is 'as good as new' if it is adequately treated and resolved, because psoriasis generally does not leave permanent scars unless patients excoriate or damage their skin in other ways. However, if the patient is afflicted with psoriatic arthritis severe enough to cause bony changes, the destruction is irreversible, even if the patient is appropriately treated at a later time with antiarthritic agents.

No topical medications are known to help psoriatic arthritis. Therefore, if early signs and symptoms appear, it is best to refer patients to a rheumatologist and prepare them for possible initiation of systemic antipsoriatic medications. In addition to improving the skin, some systemic agents can possibly slow down the destructive progression of psoriatic arthritis and are the agents of choice for those with both skin and joint manifestations.

The Koo-Menter Psoriasis Instrument (KMPI) has been developed to assist physicians in making decisions about whether the psoriasis patient can be adequately treated with topical therapy alone or whether he or she may need phototherapy or a systemic agent in addition to topical therapy (Appendix D, page 121). The KMPI is an integrated tool to help physicians perform a comprehensive evaluation of psoriasis patients including physical severity, QOL impact, and arthritis issues, and document the need for a more aggressive treatment.

Ultimately, it is a clinical judgment as to how aggressively the patient needs to be treated, and this decision should be made after taking into account all of the above-mentioned factors.

Selected Readings

Feldman SR, Koo JY, Menter A, et al: Decision points for the initiation of systemic treatment for psoriasis. *J Am Acad Dermatol* 2005;53:101-107.

Koo JY, Kowalski JW, Lebwohl MG, et al: The Koo-Menter Psoriasis Instrument for identifying candidate patients for systemic therapy. In: Koo JY, Lebwohl MG, Lee CS, eds: *Mild-to-Moderate Psoriasis*. Informa Healthcare USA, Inc, New York, NY, 2006, pp 9-28 (includes KMPI).

Chapter 5

Topical Medications for Psoriasis

F our questions a treating physician needs to ask before prescribing topical agents for psoriasis are: Which agent? Which vehicle? Which strength? Which location?

Which Agent?

The most important factor when choosing a topical medication for psoriasis is the choice between steroids and nonsteroids. There are many topical agents to consider, including topical steroids, vitamin D analogues (Dovonex®, Taclonex®), tazarotene (Tazorac®), anthralin (Psoriatec™), crude coal tar, salicylic acid, lactic acid, and nonmedicated moisturizers. Our recommendation is to concentrate on using several medications wisely, with a good understanding of appropriate patient candidates, efficacy, side effects, and expected results, rather than mastering all available topical agents. Vitamin D analogues and topical steroids are two of the most useful topical agents, especially in a primary care setting, and will be examined first. Other, more messy or perhaps less effective agents, such as anthralin, tar preparations, and tazarotene, will also be discussed.

Which Vehicle?

Topical medications are available as creams, ointments, foams, gels, lotions, liquid solutions, sprays, oils, and drug-impregnated tapes. The appropriate vehicle to use depends mostly on the location of the psoriasis as well as the patient's preference. Traditionally, it has been taught that thicker vehicles are more potent, more moisturizing, and more effective. With the same active ingredients, ointments are often stronger than creams, which are usually stronger than lotions. However, this is not always true, so it is important to study the efficacy of each individual agent. Moreover, patient preferences often take precedence as long as safety measures are heeded. Patients often appreciate a prescription for both a cream and an ointment of the same agent. Compliance with cream is best in the morning when patients feel more hurried and are thus more likely to forego their treatment. Creams spread across the skin rapidly and easily, are more quickly absorbed than ointments, and do not stain clothing. Ointments are more acceptable in the evenings, when patients have more time for application and are less concerned about the greasiness of the agent interacting with their clothing.

Twice-daily application is critically important for maximal effectiveness of most topical agents (in particular vitamin D analogues). A patient who is unhappy with a particular vehicle for practical reasons is much less likely to use the medication as directed, and will report a drug as ineffective that may actually be effective if used compliantly. This subsequently limits the available regimens and treatment options, thus forcing the physician to use higher-potency medications. Patients should be routinely encouraged to use these medications as directed so that maximal efficacy can be achieved and patients can rely less on steroids. Ask patients their opinion of their medications and try to work within these preferences to obtain maximal compliance and efficacy.

Consider the location of psoriasis when choosing a treatment vehicle. One area especially sensitive to vehicle choice is the scalp. The scalp presents a particular challenge because hair not only blocks direct application to the plaques, but also will often deter patients from using a cosmetically unsuitable medication despite its effectiveness (Figure 5-1, see color insert). Because of these factors, gels, lotions, liquid solutions, foams, and sprays are the most elegant for treating scalp psoriasis. Oils, creams, and ointments are still acceptable, and sometimes more effective, but most patients will prefer to use these at night and wash them out in the morning. One of the most important aspects of treating the scalp is to instruct the patient on appropriate application of a particular medication to ensure that it actually reaches the plaque and not just the hair. Demonstrating the application to the patient in the office with a sample is effective. Finally, be sure that patients understand that the medication must be left on the scalp, unless formulated as a shampoo. Most treatments can be applied either directly on a dry scalp, or to a damp scalp after towel drying.

Psoriasis symptoms can be another guiding factor in vehicle choice. Patients who complain of dry or itchy skin usually prefer an ointment or cream for added moisturization. Patients with fissures or cracked psoriatic plaques will complain bitterly of stinging pain if alcohol-based agents such as foams or solutions are used. Choose a nonalcohol-based medication for these patients. Gels and foams can be particularly drying and are better suited for patients who dislike the greasiness of creams and ointments, or who have oily skin.

Steroid-impregnated tape (flurandrenolide [Cordran®] tape) can be used when patients have few plaques to treat and are willing to take the time and effort to cut the tape to the appropriate size and apply it to each plaque. This is best done on extremities, where the plaques are thick, scaly, and often resistant to treatment. These areas are also more resistant to skin atrophy that can result under occlusion from steroids.

Which Strength?

Consider the location of psoriasis and disease severity before choosing a strength (Table 5-1). Next, consider the patient. Pediatric patients are more susceptible to skin thin-

Table 5-1: Ranking of Commonly Used Topical Steroids

Group	Brand Name
Class 1	Clobex® lotion
	Clobex® spray
	Clobex® shampoo
	Cormax® cr, ot
	Diprolene® gel, ot
	Psorcon® E® ot
	Temovate® cr, ot
	Ultravate® cr, ot
Class 2	Cyclocort® ot
	Diprolene® cr
	Diprosone® ot
	Elocon® ot
	Florone® ot
	Halog® cr
	Lidex® cr, gel, ot
	Psorcon® E® cr
	Topicort® cr
Class 3	Cutivate® ot
	Diprosone® cr
	Halog® ot
	Kenalog® ot
	Lidex® E cr
	Topicort® LP cr
	Valisone® ot

cr=cream; ot=ointment

Available Sizes (in grams, unless otherwise specified)	Generic Name
1 oz, 2 oz	Clobetasol propionate
2 oz, 4.25 oz	Clobetasol propionate
4 oz	Clobetasol propionate
15, 30, 45	Clobetasol propionate
15, 45	Betamethasone dipropionate
15, 30, 60	Diflorasone diacetate
15, 30, 45, 60	Clobetasol propionate
15, 50	Halobetasol propionate
15, 30, 60	Amcinonide
15, 45	Betamethasone dipropionate
15, 45	Betamethasone dipropionate
15, 45	Mometasone furoate
15, 30, 60	Diflorasone diacetate
15, 30, 60, 240	Halcinonide
15, 30, 60, 120	Fluocinonide
15, 30, 60	Diflorasone diacetate
15, 60, 4 oz	Desoximetasone
115, 30, 60	Fluticasone propionate
15, 45	Betamethasone dipropionate
15, 30, 60, 240	Halcinonide
15, 20, 60, 80	Triamcinolone acetonide
15, 30, 60, 120	Fluocinonide
15, 60	Desoximetasone
15, 45	Betamethasone valerate

(continued on next page)

Table 5-1: Ranking of Commonly Used Topical Steroids *(continued)*

Group	Brand Name
Class 4	Cordran® ot
	Cloderm® cr
	Elocon® cr
	Kenalog® cr
	Synalar® ot
	Westcort® ot
Class 5	Cordran® cr
	Cutivate® cr
	Dermatop® cr
	Locoid® cr
	Synalar® cr
	Valisone® cr
	Westcort® cr
Class 6	Capex® shampoo
	Derma-Smoothe®
	DesOwen® lotion
	DesOwen® cr
	DesOwen® ot
	Aclovate® cr, ot
	Synalar® cr
	Synalar® solution
	Tridesilon® cr, ot
Class 7	Hydrocortisone 2.5%
	Hydrocortisone 1%

cr=cream; ot=ointment; OTC=over the counter

Available Sizes (in grams, unless otherwise specified)	Generic Name
15, 30, 60	Flurandrenolide
45	Clocortolone
15, 45	Mometasone furoate
15, 60, 80	Triamcinolone acetonide
15, 30, 60	Fluocinolone acetonide
15, 45, 60	Hydrocortisone valerate
15, 30, 60	Flurandrenolide
15, 30, 60	Fluticasone propionate
15, 60	Prednicarbate
15, 45	Hydrocortisone butyrate
15, 30, 60	Fluocinolone acetonide
15, 45	Betamethasone valerate
15, 45, 60	Hydrocortisone valerate
4 oz	Fluocinolone acetonide
1 bottle	Fluocinolone
2 oz, 4 oz	Desonide
15, 60, 90	Desonide
15, 60	Desonide
15, 30, 60	Alclometasone dipropionate
15, 30, 60	Fluocinolone acetonide
20 mL, 60 mL	Fluocinolone acetonide
15, 60	Desonide
30, 60	Hydrocortisone
OTC	Hydrocortisone

ning and should be treated carefully for as short a time as possible when topical steroids are used. Elderly patients are also at higher risk, given their history of sun-damaged and inherently thinner skin. Finally, choose a strength that is conservative, but effective. Steroids are available in seven classes, ranging from over-the-counter hydrocortisone in class 7 to super-potent topical steroids in class 1.

Which Location?

The importance of considering the locations of a patient's psoriasis lies not only in matching it with the most appropriate vehicle, but also in achieving a tolerable side-effect profile, particularly when using topical steroids. The most serious side effects to be aware of when using topical steroids are skin atrophy, including striae or stretch marks, and the risk of adrenal suppression. Atrophic skin appears shiny and thin with visible underlying blood vessels and is easily traumatized (Figure 5-2, see color insert). The risk of skin atrophy varies according to the strength of topical steroid used, the anatomic location to which it is applied, and the length of time the agent is used. On nonsensitive skin, twice-daily use of a topical steroid applied focally (ie, only to the psoriatic plaques and not to unaffected skin) poses little risk of skin atrophy within 2 weeks, even with a high-strength steroid. However, after 2 weeks, the risk of skin atrophy depends on many factors, including individual variations in susceptibility among patients. Susceptibility is unpredictable; even the most experienced dermatologist cannot differentiate a susceptible patient from a resistant patient just by clinical examination. Therefore, particularly in a primary care setting, it is best to limit super-potent topical steroid use to the FDA-recommended guideline of 2 weeks continuously or less, and limit lower-strength topical steroids to the shortest possible time needed to gain control of psoriasis. After that, it is preferable to switch to a nonsteroid (ie, vitamin D analogues) for long-term maintenance.

Steroid-sensitive locations that need special consideration include the face, axilla, pannus skin folds, inner thighs, and groin. These are high-risk areas because they tend to have thinner skin and, in the case of the axilla, groin, and inframammary and abdominal pannus skin folds, create a natural occlusion, which can increase topical potency. This makes the area more susceptible to adverse side effects, especially steroid-induced atrophy, striae, telangiectasias, and erythema.

Patients are at greater risk of developing these complications if they were inadequately counseled on appropriate use and potential side effects of topical steroids. This is one of the most common reasons for dermatologic lawsuits. Physicians need to stress proper usage to avoid these distressing situations. Striae are usually the most distressing adverse reaction because of their unsightliness and irreversibility (Figure 5-3, see color insert).

If steroids must be used in high-risk areas, physicians may first try those from classes 5, 6, or 7. Topical steroids from class 4 are usually the highest potency acceptable for long-term use in steroid-sensitive areas. Whether for regular strength or steroid-sensitive areas, the use of a stronger topical steriod should be limited over time with the intent of transitioning patients to other, safer topical agents. One pitfall in primary care dermatology is that patients are often instructed appropriately on limiting their steroid use, but then are not given a transition or tapering regimen to follow. This leaves many patients in the trap of treating their disease for 2 weeks and achieving some satisfying results, and then abruptly discontinuing treatment only to see the disease flare again. This vacillating regimen is both frustrating and unproductive, and can be eliminated by the use of sequential therapy (see Chapter 9).

Steroids should also be used carefully on the face. Facial skin is thin and sensitive. Beside skin atrophy, it is at high risk for topical steroid complications such as perioral dermatitis, steroid-induced acne, folliculitis, rosacea, hypertrichosis, and hypopigmentation. Again, patients are less tolerant of these side effects because of the cosmetic sensitivity of the area. They should be treated cautiously after adequate counseling. The risk of adverse side effects, however, should be balanced with the severity of disease. If the patient's psoriasis is disfiguring and distressing because of its location, it is worth treating more aggressively with close supervision to improve the patient's quality of life (QOL).

Optimal Use of Topical Steroids for Psoriasis

Psoriasis is thought to be only moderately responsive to topical steroids. Therefore, to obtain an adequate response, the physician needs to use a stronger steroid than what is typically used when treating other common, chronic inflammatory conditions such as eczema or seborrheic dermatitis.

Topical steroid use in psoriasis is also well known to be associated with tachyphylaxis, a phenomenon in which the medications initially work well, but efficacy gradually diminishes with continuous use. In time, topical steroids may become useless. To regain effectiveness, the physician needs to increase steroid potency or give the patient a 'steroid holiday' lasting several months. This drawback has led to the development of intermittent treatment, or pulse therapy, whereby patients use nonsteroid medications such as vitamin D analogues throughout the week, and steroids only on weekends (see Chapter 9). This approach can be followed long term even with high-potency steroids as long as patients are compliant with the alternating regimen and periodically monitored for side effects.

Steroid strengths typically used for psoriasis range from midstrength agents such as triamcinolone (Kenalog®) 0.1% cream or 0.1% ointment, which are class 4 and 3 respectively, to high-strength agents such as fluocinonide ointment (Lidex®), which is class 2, or mometasone cream or ointment (Elocon®), which is class 4 as a cream or lotion and class 2 as an ointment. Class 1, or super-potent topical steroids such as clobetasol (Temovate® cream or ointment, Clobex® spray), or halobetasol (Ultravate® cream or ointment), are the highest-strength steroids available and are often needed for thick, scaly psoriasis. Topical steroids that are weaker than midstrength generally are not adequately effective for plaque-type psoriasis, especially in nonsensitive areas such as the extremities, where plaques tend to be more resistant.

Physicians should use the lowest possible steroid strength that the patient feels is adequate and the physician believes to be safe. The US Food and Drug Administration (FDA) recommends that class 1 steroids such as clobetasol or halobetasol be used for no more than 2 to 4 weeks at a time (depending on the formulation) to avoid skin atrophy and adrenal suppression. Longer use requires closer supervision. Whenever topical steroids must be discontinued, they should be tapered off rather than abruptly stopped because abrupt discontinuation may lead to a rebound phenomenon. In this rare phenomenon, psoriasis suddenly becomes even more inflamed than at pretreatment baseline after sudden discontinuation of the steroid. The risk of rebound is greater if there is no replacement therapy offered; the risk can be minimized with a follow-through therapy, such as with a nonsteroid agent.

The amount of class 1 steroid applied each week should also be limited to avoid risk of adrenal suppression. Adrenal suppression may occur with any of the midstrength to super-potent topical steroids. Patients at higher risk include infants and children who have a high skin surface-to-body mass ratio and patients with extensive psoriasis who use large quantities of the drug. For super-potent topical steroids, adult patients should use no more than 2 oz (ie, 50 to 60 g)/week.

In summary, topical steroids are best suited for a 'quick-fix' or rapid improvement of psoriasis when the patient first presents.

Calcipotriene (Dovonex®) Cream and Calcitriol (Vectical®) Ointment

One of the most important features of a vitamin D analogue that makes it an excellent agent for primary care physicians as well as for dermatologists is its safety profile. Vitamin D analogues are steroid-free, and thus free from steroid side effects such as skin thinning, striae formation, and adrenal suppression. Most skin cells possess a nuclear receptor for vitamin D, which has been shown to be responsible for decreasing cellular proliferation and increasing cellular differentiation. For these reasons, vitamin D can be helpful in battling psoriasis. Calcipotriene (Dovonex®) and calcitriol (Vectical®) are topical vitamin D_3 analogues modified to minimize the systemic side effects affecting calcium levels. They are the first elegant nonsteroidal alternatives for the treatment of psoriasis.

The primary adverse side effect of calcipotriene is lesional and perilesional (around the lesion) irritation. Irritation from calcipotriene usually presents with a red ring of inflamed skin surrounding the treated lesions (Figure 5-4, see color insert). Patients report a mild stinging or burning sensation. This is usually transient, and patients quickly become accustomed to it. The irritation is usually more pronounced on the face and occluded parts of the body such as axilla and groin. It appears to depend largely on the penetration of calcipotriene through the skin. The skin-to-skin occlusion inherent in the axilla and groin enhances penetration of calcipotriene, which is thought to account for the increased rate of irritation in these areas. Calcipotriene also is lipophilic and more readily absorbed by skin containing oily sebaceous glands, such as the face, which also helps explain why it tends to be more irritating on the face. In fact, for this reason, per package insert, neither calcipotriene cream nor calcitriol ointment are allowed to be used on the face.

The systemic adverse side effect to be aware of when using calcipotriene is hypercalcemia. Hypercalcemia has been reported only in rare instances when a patient has used large amounts of this medication on the body. The FDA label includes the need to limit total weekly use of calcipotriene in all formulations (ie, cream, solution) to 100 g/wk. The limit for calcitriol ointment (Vectical®) is 200 g/wk.

Twice-daily application of calcipotriene ointment has been shown in two randomized, double-blind, multicenter studies to be more effective than the use of high-strength topical steroid ointment (ie, fluocinonide) twice daily. However, this result was seen only if the patient used calcipotriene consistently twice a day, every day. If subjects were noncompliant, they were withdrawn from the study. These stringent criteria probably had much to do with the success of the medication. The efficacy of once-daily calcipotriene is approximately half that of twice-daily use during the first month of use, while the efficacy of fluocinonide used once a day is only mildly inferior than twice a day.

Patients need to be well educated when they are given a prescription for calcipotriene. If the patient is to use calcipotriene as monotherapy, it is critical to communicate the importance of using it twice a day and warn of possible skin irritation. However, the most effective formulation of calcipotriene, calcipotriene ointment, is no longer available in the US. Only the less effective cream formulation is still available.

A new vitamin D agent, calcitriol ointment (Vectical®), has been approved in the US for the treatment of plaque psoriasis. Calcitriol, the naturally occurring hormonally active form of vitamin D_3, is an effective topical psoriasis medication with a strong safety profile in long-term treatment. Topical calcitriol 3 μg/g ointment was superior to vehicle ointment alone in two randomized, double-blind clinical trials. In a long-term, 1-year, open-label study, calcitriol produced steady continued improvement in psoriatic lesions for the entire time period, with a low risk of adverse events and without reported clinical effects on systemic calcium homeostasis. In a direct right-to-left bilateral comparison of calcipotriene ointment and calcitriol ointment, the latter produced greater improvement of psoriasis lesions on flexural skin areas with a lower incidence of skin irritation and was preferred by patients. As with calcipotriene, patient education for calcitriol ointment is key to compliance.

Calcipotriene/Betamethasone Dipropionate (Taclonex®) Ointment

A combination calcipotriene (0.005%)/betamethasone dipropionate (0.064%) ointment (Taclonex®) for psoriasis available in the US has a betamethasone dipropionate component that is is roughly equivalent to high-strength rather than super-potent topical steroids. This agent works just as well once a day as twice a day. The skin irritation rate of the calcipotriene/betamethasone dipropionate combination is much less than calcipotriene ointment used alone. In various clinical trials involving >2,000 patients, the calcipotriene/betamethasone dipropionate combination was noted to decrease the average Psoriasis Area and Severity Index (PASI) by 50% to 70% within the first 3 weeks. Moreover, because this agent works well once a day, patients can cover twice the area with the same amount of medication, time, and effort compared with other topical antipsoriasis agents, which usually require twice daily application for up to 4-6 weeks to achieve maximum efficacy. Lastly, compliance with this combination medication may be better than with the traditional topical agents because of once-a-day dosing and the absence of heightened concerns regarding side effects that are typically associated with the use of super-potent topical steroids.

In a 52-week study conducted from August 2002 to April 2004, 634 patients were randomized, double-blind, to treatment (once daily, when required) with either 52 weeks of Taclonex®, 52 weeks of alternating 4-week periods of Taclonex® and calcipotriene monotherapy, or 4 weeks of Taclonex® followed by 48 weeks of calcipotriene alone. The severity of psoriasis was moderate in 69.1% of patients, severe in 27.9%, and very severe in 3%. The median duration rate of psoriasis was 17 years (range=1 to 65 years).

In previous short-term, 4-week studies, the efficacy of the combination ointment was found to be superior to the use of calcipotriene alone. The current study showed that the efficacy of the combination ointment used for up to 52 weeks was consistently better than 4 weeks of its use followed by 48 weeks of calcipotriene use alone, or aternating a 4-week regimen between the 2 agents. Moreover, there were no reported cases of hypothalamic/pituitary/adrenal (HPA) axis suppression or striae in the combination group despite the fact that >200 subjects used the combination agent for 52 weeks. Less than 2% of this group was noted to have skin atrophy other than striae. Lastly, the combination group had the least problem with skin irritation compared with the other two groups. Currently, Taclonex® is approved by the FDA for the topical treatment of psoriasis vulgaris in adults 18 years of age and above for up to 4 weeks.

Other Topical Agents

Other topical agents that may be less effective, require extra caution, or involve special instructions are described in the sections that follow. Potential problems can result because they may be messier or more difficult to use because of their side effect profiles. However, with appropriate knowledge and training, they can be excellent resources when treating psoriasis while avoiding the dangers of excessive reliance on topical steroids.

Tazarotene

Tazarotene (Tazorac®) is a topical retinoid (modified vitamin A) that was first approved for plaque-type psoriasis in the US in 1997, and is now also approved for acne and fine-wrinkle reduction. It is available in a cream in 0.05% and 0.1% strengths and a gel in 0.05% and 0.1% strengths. The gel tends to be more elegant, spread more rapidly, and absorb more quickly, making it good for large surfaces as well as for the scalp. The cream is more moisturizing, and, therefore, more appropriate for nonscalp application.

Tazarotene can be effective as a single agent used once daily, but is often used in combination with topical steroids. Patients who use tazarotene as a monotherapy should apply the medication to the plaques once daily in the evenings, taking care to avoid the surrounding skin.

The most frequently reported adverse reactions of tazarotene are similar to and more commonly reported than those of calcipotriene, including lesional and perilesional irritation, burning, stinging, itching, and redness. Many patients find tazarotene irritating. These patients should be placed on the lower strength. A second option is to decrease the frequency of application to every other day or every third day.

Although tazarotene is effective when used alone, most dermatologists combine it with another agent. According to the package insert, tazarotene should be avoided with concomitant dermatologic medications and cosmetics that have a strong drying effect.

A final note to remember about tazarotene when prescribing it in the US is that it is pregnancy Category X. Caution should be taken when using this drug in women of child-bearing age based on the risk associated with oral retinoids. Patients should be counseled, have a pregnancy test before starting therapy, and use adequate contraception during treatment.

Anthralin

Because of its moderate efficacy, risk of irritation, and overall messiness, anthralin is one of the less commonly used agents in the US. It is less effective than twice-daily calcipotriene, but can still be a useful agent in some patients who do not respond to vitamin D analogues or tazarotene. Most commonly, it is used in a day-care setting as described by the Ingram regimen, using UVB phototherapy followed by all day application of anthralin. Anthralin can also be used at home by motivated patients who fail or do not tolerate other topical treatments or who need to avoid steroids.

One disadvantage of anthralin treatment to warn patients about is the inevitable purplish, brownish staining of clothing, porcelain, and skin (Figure 5-5, see color insert). A newer formulation, 1% anthralin, is formulated with a temperature-sensitive vehicle that releases active medication when applied to skin. It shows comparable efficacy with less staining, especially if cool water without soap is used to wash it off. Most patients are willing to tolerate these nuisances to alleviate their symptoms and can be reassured that skin staining disappears several weeks after discontinuing treatment. The most important adverse reaction is skin irritation, usually occurring days after the first application (Figure 5-6, see color insert). This mostly occurs on uninvolved skin, so patients should try to apply the thick paste with a tongue depressor only to the plaques. Some overlap onto normal surrounding skin is unavoidable, but this often fades with continued use (Figure 5-7, see color insert).

Short-contact therapy remains the most efficacious way to treat patients who are irritated by the medication. Anthralin is preferentially absorbed by psoriatic plaques, and most of the absorption occurs within the first hour of application. Therefore, applying the medication for 30 minutes to 1 hour before bathing reduces the risk of irritation as well as staining, while maintaining efficacy. Patients should follow with a moisturizing emollient. Phototherapy as well as other topical or oral treatments can be used in combination with anthralin for maximal efficacy.

Coal-Tar Preparations

Compared with other psoriasis treatments, tar remains one of the safest. The FDA ruled that there is no convincing evidence of carcinogenic risk with human therapeutic use of coal tar in concentration up to 5%.

Messiness is one major obstacle when using tar. Old pajamas and bedclothes should be used during this treatment. Side effects of tar products include skin irritation, folliculitis, photosensitivity, and exacerbation of pustular psoriasis.

Coal tar is a mixture of at least 10,000 components, most of which have not been identified. It comes from the distillation of coal in the absence of oxygen. Crude coal tar in combination with phototherapy in a day-care setting is still the most effective treatment available for moderate-to-severe psoriasis since it was first described by Goeckerman in 1925. Coal-tar preparations have some of the longest track records for face usage in actual patients. They can be applied to the entire body on both normal and abnormal skin. Tar products are available in many different formulations and strengths (Table 5-2). Getting a good history from the patient will allow the physician to tailor the regimen to the type and location of psoriasis, and to any personal specifications the patient may have.

Brown tar or gold tar is called liquor carbonis detergens (LCD) and can be made in concentrations of up to 20% blended in multiple different vehicles. It is a weak formulation and, therefore, should be prescribed in the higher strength, unless skin intolerance dictates the need for a lower strength. It can be applied to the skin as a leave-on moisturizer multiple times per day, used in bath water for tar soaks, or used to saturate the scalp under shower-cap occlusion. Patients can achieve added benefit by applying the medication in the evening and occluding it with plastic wrap for increased potency and effectiveness. Brown tar is also available as various FDA-approved, over-the-counter preparations such as tar shampoos and tar soaks.

Black tar is a thick, crude coal-tar product in petrolatum base that can be formulated in 2%, 5%, and 10% strengths. It is primarily used in day-care settings (see Chapter 8), but patients who do not mind the inconvenience can achieve

Table 5-2: Commonly Used Tar Preparations

Brown or Gold Tar

5% LCD	In Nutraderm® lotion
10% LCD	In Nutraderm® lotion
20% LCD	In Nutraderm® lotion

Black Tar

2% crude coal tar	In petrolatum (ointment)
5% crude coal tar	In petrolatum (ointment)
10% crude coal tar	In petrolatum (ointment)
2% crude coal tar	In nonionic base (cream)

LCD=liquor carbonis detergens

success with home use. They should be encouraged to apply the medication in a downward motion in line with the growth of their hair follicles to decrease the risk of developing folliculitis. Plastic wrap can be used to occlude the tar and reduce soaking into clothing. The tar should be left on for at least 4 hours for maximum efficacy, and many patients complete this regimen at night while sleeping. Mineral oil application followed by bathing and shampooing should be used to remove the medication.

Salicylic Acid

Keratolytics act to remove excess scale and hyperkeratosis associated with psoriasis. They are available in many different vehicles in strengths ranging from 2% to 20%. Keratolytics can be used on scaly patches on the body as well as on thick, adherent scalp psoriasis. These med-

Table 5-3: Maximal Scalp Treatment Using Salicylic Acid (Keralyt® Gel, Salex® Lotion), and Tar Preparation

At Bedtime:

- Apply Keralyt® gel to scaly areas of scalp.

- Apply 20% tar preparation, using squeeze bottle with tip applicator, to entire scalp by parting hair in 0.5-inch sections and massaging medication in with fingers.

- Cover with shower cap. Place stocking cap or cut thigh section of ladies' nylon stocking over shower cap for better occlusion throughout the night.

In the Morning:

- During the morning shower, gently massage scales and medication out of hair with Neutrogena® T/Gel® Shampoo Extra Strength or similar tar preparation.

- Towel dry hair after showering.

- Apply any options of tazarotene gel, calcipotriene scalp solution, and steroid solution or foam to damp scalp, taking care to apply medication directly to scalp rather than hair.

- Style hair as usual.

- In the evening, several hours before starting the regimen again, apply second dose of calcipotriene scalp solution and/or topical steroid to achieve twice-daily application.

---

ications are functional only as 'descaling' agents. They do not affect erythema or induration, and therefore should be used simultaneously with other topical agents. Patients and Goeckerman day-care centers often mix keratolytics with tar products. One agent that should not be used simultaneously with acidic products is calcipotriene. Calcipotriene is a fragile molecule easily destroyed by acidic pH. However, the two agents can be used sequentially as long as application is separated by at least 2 hours. Salicylic acid is the most commonly used keratolytic agent and is commercially available over the counter as 6% Keralyt® gel or Salex® lotion. The gel formulation makes it a convenient, easily applied scalp therapy. An excellent regimen using a salicylic acid agent is described in Table 5-3.

Salicylic acid can produce local irritation and erythema, especially on normal skin surrounding the psoriatic plaques. In addition, indiscriminate use can lead to excessive systemic absorption, causing salicylism. Symptoms of salicylism include nausea, tinnitus, and hyperventilation. Systemic absorption of salicylic acid can also inhibit gluconeogenesis and lead to hypoglycemia in diabetics. Other agents such as lactic acid should be used for this population.

Selected Readings

Ashton RE, Lowe NJ: Anthralin therapy of psoriasis. In: Lowe NJ, ed: *Practical Psoriasis Therapy,* 2nd ed. St. Louis, MO, Mosby-Year Book, 1993, pp 59-71.

Bowman PH, Maloney JE, Koo JY: Combination of calcipotriene (Dovonex) ointment and tazarotene (Tazorac) gel versus clobetasol ointment in the treatment of plaque psoriasis: a pilot study. *J Am Acad Dermatol* 2002;46:907-913.

Bruce S, Epinette WW, Funicella T, et al: Comparative study of calcipotriene (MC903) ointment and fluocinonide ointment in the treatment of psoriasis. *J Am Acad Dermatol* 1994;31:755-759.

Callis KP, Krueger GG: Topical agents in the treatment of moderate-to-severe psoriasis. In: Weinstein GD, Gottlieb AB, eds: *Therapy of Moderate-to-Severe Psoriasis*, 2nd ed. New York, NY, Marcel Dekker, 2003, pp 29-51.

Christophers E, Mroweitz U: Psoriasis. In: Fitzpatrick TB, Freedberg IM, Eisen AZ, et al, eds: *Dermatology in General Medicine,* 5th ed. New York, NY, McGraw-Hill, 1999, pp 495-533.

Cornell RC, Stoughton RB: Topical steroids. In: Lowe NJ, ed: *Practical Psoriasis Therapy,* 2nd ed. St. Louis, MO, Mosby-Year Book, 1993, pp 33-43.

Goeckerman WH: The treatment of psoriasis. *Northwest Med* 1981;24:229-231.

Gribetz C, Ling M, Lebwohl M, et al: Pimecrolimus cream 1% in the treatment of intertriginous psoriasis: a double-blind, randomized study. *J Am Acad Dermatol* 2004;51:731-738.

Hecker DJ, Lebwohl M: Clinical experience with vitamin D analogues. In: Roenigk HH, Maibach HI, eds: *Psoriasis,* 3rd ed. New York, NY, Marcel Dekker, 1998, pp 507-510.

Koo J, Siebenlist J, et al: Vitamin D analogues in the treatment of psoriasis. In: Roenigk HH, Maibach HI, eds: *Psoriasis,* 3rd ed. New York, NY, Marcel Dekker, 1998, pp 497-506.

Koo JY, Lebwohl MG, Lee CS, eds: *Mild-to-Moderate Psoriasis.* Informa Healthcare USA, Inc, New York, NY, 2006.

Kraft S, Maibach HI, et al: Dithranol (Anthralin). In: Roenigk HH, Maibach HI, eds: *Psoriasis,* 3rd ed. New York, NY, Marcel Dekker, 1998, pp 435-452.

Kragballe K, Austad J, Barnes L, et al: Efficacy results of a 52-week, randomised, double-blind, safety study of a calcipotriol/betamethasone dipropionate two-compound product (Daivobet/Dovobet/Taclonex) in the treatment of psoriasis vulgaris. *Dermatology* 2006;213:319-326.

Kragballe K, Austad J, Barnes L, et al: A 52-week randomized safety study of a calcipotriol/betamethasone dipropionate two-compound product (Dovobet/Daivobet/Taclonex) in the treatment of psoriasis vulgaris. *Br J Dermatol* 2006;154:1155-1160.

Kragballe K, van de Kerkhof PC: Consistency of data in six phase III clinical studies of a two-compound product containing calcipotriol and betamethasone dipropionate ointment for the treatment of psoriasis. *J Eur Acad Dermatol Venereol* 2006;20:39-44.

Lebwohl M, Freeman AK, Chapman MS, et al: Tacrolimus ointment is effective for facial and intertriginous psoriasis. *J Am Acad Dermatol* 2004;51:723-730.

Lowe NJ: Tars, keratolytics, and emollients. In: Lowe NJ, ed: *Practical Psoriasis Therapy,* 2nd ed. St. Louis, MO, Mosby-Year Book, 1993, pp 45-57.

Ranking of topical steroids. Galderma Laboratories Inc, Fort Worth, TX, 1999.

Steele JA, Choi C, Kwong PC: Topical tacrolimus in the treatment of inverse psoriasis in children. *J Am Acad Dermatol* 2005;53: 713-716.

5

Chapter 6

Phototherapy

Phototherapy, or the repeated use of ultraviolet light to treat skin disease, is one of the oldest known treatments for psoriasis. It is effective for generalized psoriasis as well as for severe hand and foot psoriasis. Patients can receive treatment either in their dermatologist's office in an outpatient setting or, in some cases, in the comfort and convenience of their own homes. Phototherapy can be accomplished in a standup booth, in front of a standing light panel, with single panels for hands or feet only, or with handheld wands (Figure 6-1, see color insert). The three most common types of phototherapy use ultraviolet A (UVA) wavelengths, ultraviolet B (UVB) wavelengths, or a focused spectrum of UVB called narrow-band UVB (Table 6-1). Examining the methods and principles of phototherapy is beyond the scope of this text. Only general facts will be covered here.

UVB phototherapy includes wavelengths between 290 and 320 nm on the electromagnetic spectrum. Because of its extensive use during the past century and its long track record of safety and efficacy, UVB phototherapy continues to enjoy widespread use. The versatility of UVB adds to its attractiveness. It can be combined with almost any other treatment modality, including topical, oral, and biologic, for greater efficacy. UVB phototherapy is usually reserved to treat psoriasis that is unresponsive to topical medications or too widespread to make twice-daily topical application a feasible option.

If a patient has >10% of their total body surface area involved (1% is approximately equal to the surface area of the

Table 6-1: Types of Phototherapy

Phototherapy	Procedure
• UVB	290-320 nm
• Laser narrow-band UVB	308 nm
• Narrow-band UVB	311-312 nm
• Oral PUVA	320-400 nm with oral psoralen

PUVA=psoralen plus ultraviolet A; UVB=ultraviolet B

patient's palm and thumb), treatment with topical therapy alone is difficult; the patient is likely to need phototherapy and/or systemic therapy in addition to topical agents.

When initiating phototherapy, patients should be treated three times per week. This regimen can later be tapered and eventually maintained at a low frequency or discontinued altogether, but some busy patients find this schedule difficult. In these cases, home light can be an alternative for a reliable and compliant patient.

Side effects and contraindications to phototherapy include burning and photosensitivity reactions. One logistic disadvantage is the extensive time commitment required for this treatment, in addition to three times a week insurance copayments.

Narrow-band UVB is a newer technique that uses a narrower spectrum of energy thought to be most effective for psoriasis clearance. In the US, narrow-band UVB is steadily replacing broad-band UVB as the predominant form of UVB phototherapy. One reason for its popularity is that it has been shown to be more effective than broad-band UVB. Available long-term data has revealed no convincing evidence that therapeutic broad-band or narrow-band UVB increases the risk of skin cancer. However, for narrow-band UVB, the database is still several decades old, as opposed to broad-band UVB, for which there is nearly one century worth of worldwide human experience.

Psoralen plus UVA (PUVA) uses a photosensitizing medication taken orally or absorbed topically in combination with UVA phototherapy. PUVA penetrates more deeply into the tissue than broad-band UVB or narrow-band UVB, is more effective than its UVB counterparts, and provides a longer remission. After 30 years of use, PUVA continues to be one of the best psoriasis treatments available, especially for recalcitrant or widespread cases of psoriasis, including thick lesions found on palms and soles.

Like UVB, PUVA requires a time commitment at least initially, but can be tapered to a maintenance regimen as infrequent as once per month in patients who achieve a complete remission. Such results can dramatically change the life of a suffering patient. However, PUVA also has its own complications, such as nausea, headaches, dizziness (when taken orally), burning, itching, and photosensitivity. Proven in Caucasian patients only, it has been shown that PUVA increases the risk of developing squamous cell skin cancer. Controversy continues about whether or not it increases the risk of melanoma with long-term use. Thus far, one large-scale study showed an increased risk of melanoma only after 15 years of follow-up, and mainly in those who had at least 250 PUVA treatments. An even larger long-term study from Sweden showed no increased risk of melanoma with PUVA. Approximately 20 other published studies with smaller cohorts and/or shorter follow-up periods failed to demonstrate increased risk of melanoma. Squamous cell carcinoma and melanomas are relevant issues primarily for fair-skinned individuals or for those patients who have had at least 200 to 250 treatment sessions.

Laser therapy (fiberoptically-directed monochromatic UVB light) is another newer form of phototherapy that targets only psoriatic plaques. This allows more aggressive phototherapy compared to traditional UVB and PUVA, which exposes noninvolved skin as well as psoriatic skin to UV light. With aggressive excimer laser therapy, psoriasis can improve significantly or clear in approximately 10 sessions instead of the 30 to 40 sessions needed with regular full-body phototherapy. This dramatic difference is because psoriatic lesions are able to withstand a much higher dose of light than noninvolved skin. Excimer laser therapy dosing is determined by the maximum tolerance of *psoriatic* skin, whereas traditional full-body UV therapy dosing is determined by the minimal erythema dose (MED) of *noninvolved* skin. MED refers to the amount of light exposure that results in the induction of barely perceptible erythema on the noninvolved skin; it is the traditional limit on how aggressively nonlaser phototherapy can be conducted (UVB doses beyond the MED will burn the patient).

Delivery of higher doses than MED are made possible with targeted UV application with the laser and results in faster clinical response and greater clinical efficacy. The supraerythemogenic phototherapy strategy involves delivering UVB at a dose much greater than the MED. This is in contrast to the traditional phototherapy options that were either erythemogenic (ie, at MED) or suberythemogenic (ie, just below MED) strategy for conducting phototherapy. Instead of being limited by the MED, supraerythemogenic laser phototherapy can be conducted much more aggressively; it is only limited by the minimal blistering dose (MBD), which is the lowest dose of laser narrow-band UVB irradiation that results in blistering of the psoriatic lesions. More precisely, the optimal laser dosage is sub-MBD dose (ie, dosimetry just below the MBD). Hence, the new supraerythemogenic phototherapy strategy with laser results in a fewer number of sessions needed for clearance. In short, laser phototherapy has much more efficacy than traditional UVB phototherapy, and the onset of action is much faster because physicians can go considerably beyond MED in aggressiveness of dosimetry.

In addition, excimer laser therapy results in no photo damage to noninvolved skin, given its targeted application. The Photomedex XTRAC® Velocity is the latest version of the excimer laser, which is 300% to 400% more powerful than its predecessor, the XTRAC® Ultra machine. This increased power makes treatment of generalized, moderate to severe psoriasis not only feasible but attractive. Time required for each treatment is decreased by one-third, compared to the XTRAC® Ultra, which was previously the most powerful excimer laser machine. With XTRAC® Velocity, it is expected that *generalized* psoriasis patients with 10% to 20% total body surface involvement can be treated in 10-15 min and marked improvement can be achieved after approximately 10 laser treatment sessions.

One important point to remember when caring for a patient receiving phototherapy is the interaction of light with other medications. The list of photosensitizing drugs is extensive; common offenders include thiazide diuretics, loop diuretics, antibiotics, antidepressants, and antipsychotics. Use of these medications is not prohibited, but communication about them is essential. Treating physicians and nurses must be aware of photosensitizing medications, especially when they are initiated midtreatment, so that dosimetry can be adjusted accordingly to avoid burning patients or precipitating a phototoxic reaction (ie, burn).

Finally, for patients who are unable to tolerate phototherapy, heliotherapy may be an option, especially in darker skin types. Heliotherapy is the purposeful, methodical exposure to sunlight or tanning beds. All patients should be instructed on safe methods of exposure.

Selected Readings

Gattu S, Pang ML, Pugashetti R, et al: Pilot evaluation of supra-erythemogenic phototherapy with excimer laser in the treatment of patients with moderate to severe plaque psoriasis. *J Dermatolog Treat* 2010; 21:54-60.

Hong J, Malick F, Sivanesan P, et al: Expanding use of the 308nm excimer laser for treatment of psoriasis. *Practical Dermatol* 2007;(suppl):April: 13-16.

Koo JY, Bandow G, et al: The art and practice of UVB phototherapy for the treatment of psoriasis. In: Weinstein GD, Gottlieb AB, eds: *Therapy of Moderate-to-Severe Psoriasis*, 2nd ed. New York, NY, Marcel Dekker, 2003, pp 53-90.

Lindelof B, Sigurgeirsson B, Tegner E, et al: PUVA and cancer risk: the Swedish follow-up study. *Br J Dermatol* 1999;141:108-112.

Morison WL: Systemic and topical PUVA therapy. In: Weinstein GD, Gottlieb AB, eds: *Therapy of Moderate-to-Severe Psoriasis*, 2nd ed. New York, NY, Marcel Dekker, 2003, pp 91-114.

Stern RS, Nichols KT, Vakeva LH: Malignant melanoma in patients treated for psoriasis with methoxsalen (psoralen) and ultraviolet A radiation (PUVA). The PUVA Follow-Up Study. *N Engl J Med* 1997;336:1041-1045.

6

Chapter 7

Oral Agents

Systemic Corticosteroids

Systemic corticosteroids are not indicated for the treatment of psoriasis and should be avoided whenever possible. Although they are effective in improving psoriatic lesions, patients will quickly relapse and can experience severe rebound upon discontinuation. Rebound occurs when patients develop even larger areas of psoriasis than before they began treatment or when the characteristics of their disease change to a more serious form of psoriasis (eg, conversion from plaque-type to erythrodermic or pustular psoriasis). The eruption that occurs after withdrawal from treatment with systemic corticosteroids is often more recalcitrant to treatment than the initial disease. Of course, a patient may require systemic corticosteroids for treatment of a concomitant medical condition (eg, asthma or arthritis exacerbation). Be aware of the potential for psoriasis rebound upon cessation of the medication.

Patients will likely need to be tapered slowly and closely monitored for rebound.

Methotrexate

Methotrexate (Trexall™) was approved by the US Food and Drug Administration (FDA) for use in psoriasis in the early 1970s. Originally, methotrexate was thought to slow the pathologic increase in the rate of cell replication found in psoriatic skin by interfering with DNA synthesis. However, methotrexate most likely acts through an immunosuppressive rather than an antiproliferative mechanism.

Methotrexate should be avoided in patients with renal, hepatic, or hematologic abnormalities. Patients with a history of alcohol abuse should not use methotrexate because hepatotoxicity is associated with long-term exposure to alcohol. In the absence of risk factors for liver disease, a baseline liver biopsy is not necessary before starting methotrexate. In patients with persistently abnormal liver function tests (LFTs) or risk factors for hepatic disease, a pretreatment liver biopsy is required. Methotrexate is teratogenic and Category X, and women should not conceive, nor should men impregnate anyone, while they are taking the drug and for 3 months following the last dose. This medication also carries several black box warnings, including an increased risk of lymphoma and methotrexate-induced pneumonitis.

Before initiating therapy, certain tests, including baseline renal function tests, liver function tests, hepatitis screening, and a complete blood count (CBC), should be performed to ensure no contraindications are present. Also, according to the package insert, a baseline chest x-ray should be obtained to rule out lung disease or pneumonitis before starting therapy. If these laboratory tests are within normal limits, a test dose of 2.5 mg to 5 mg is typically given to assess tolerability and safety. Laboratory tests should be repeated several days after taking the test dose, and the patient should be asked about any side effects. The most common symptoms reported with the use of methotrexate include nausea, vomiting, malaise, and headache. An antiemetic can be added, if needed. Folic acid can also be added to help with gastrointestinal symptoms, although there is controversy about whether or not folic acid decreases the efficacy of methotrexate in psoriasis.

More serious adverse reactions to be aware of are bone marrow suppression, hepatotoxicity, and pneumonitis, which are rare. Additionally, patients can develop acute photosensitivity after starting methotrexate. This is especially relevant in patients undergoing concomitant phototherapy. Light therapy should not be given for at least 24 hours after the administration of methotrexate. Generally, the severity of side effects is dose-related, and methotrexate can be titrated to maximize efficacy while minimizing adverse side effects. The usual dose required for good clearing in a nonelderly adult patient is 15 mg/wk taken in three divided doses, 8 to 12 hours apart; a typical maximum dose of up to 30 mg/wk can be given. Laboratory tests should be considered. For example, according to the package insert, hematology tests should be repeated every month and renal/liver tests should be repeated every 1-2 months while on treatment. Also, the package insert states that the usual recommendation is to obtain a liver biopsy at (1) pretherapy or shortly after initiation of therapy (2-4 months), (2) after a total cumulative dose of 1.5 g, and (3) after each additional 1-1.5 g.

While a dermatologist or rheumatologist will most often be the prescribing and monitoring physician for methotrexate, the primary care physician needs to be aware of potential drug interactions that may occur while caring for the psoriasis patient on methotrexate. Trimethoprim (found in Bactrim® and Septra®), in combination with methotrexate, can cause severe bone marrow suppression and should never be given concomitantly. Barbiturates, probenecid (Probalan®), phenytoin (Dilantin®, Phenytek®), sulfonamides, and some nonsteroidal anti-inflammatory drugs (NSAIDs) can increase the serum level or half-life of methotrexate through various mechanisms. Physicians should carefully check the manufacturer's prescribing information for a complete list of drug interactions.

Cyclosporine

Cyclosporine (Gengraf®, Neoral®, Sandimmune®) works, in part, by inhibiting T-cell production of interleukin-2 (IL-2), a cytokine that plays a key role in activating T cells and propagating the inflammatory cascade.

According to the package insert, cyclosporine is usually reserved for patients with severe, recalcitrant psoriasis who have failed one other systemic therapy. At a higher dosage range (ie, 4 mg/kg/d), the effects of cyclosporine are rapid and dramatic compared with the slower onset of action of other psoriasis treatments. While liver toxicity is the major concern with methotrexate, the kidney is the main organ for toxicity concern with cyclosporine. Patients need to be closely monitored for the development of nephrotoxicity and hypertension, and cyclosporine should be avoided in patients with baseline renal dysfunction.

Patients who are considered for cyclosporine therapy must be free of serious infection, immunosuppressive states (eg, human immunodeficiency virus [HIV]), and current signs or a history of malignancy. Malignancies have been reported in transplant patients who have received cyclosporine for an extended period at doses two to three times those used in dermatology. However, studies have failed to show any convincing evidence for an increase in internal cancers, including lymphoma, in psoriasis patients whose treatment with cyclosporine followed dermatologic guidelines. Some data suggest a slight-to-moderate increase in nonmelanoma skin cancer risk, which may primarily be of concern to Caucasion people who have had previous exposure to psoralen plus ultraviolet A (PUVA) phototherapy. Cyclosporine should be used cautiously in patients with a long history of treatment with PUVA because they already have an increased risk of developing skin cancer. According to the package insert, cyclosporine should not be used concomitantly with PUVA, UVB phototherapy, or coal tar preparations.

Before initiating therapy, two baseline blood pressure readings, at least a day apart, should be obtained. Additionally, the following laboratory tests must be performed: renal function tests and liver function tests with two creatinine measurements at least a day apart, magnesium and potassium levels, a CBC, a fasting lipid profile, and uric acid level. If these results are within normal limits, cyclosporine can be started at a dosage of 2.5 mg/kg/d and titrated upward by 0.5 mg/kg/d every month to a maximum of 4 mg/kg/d. Ideal body weight should be used to avoid overdosing in patients who are obese. According to the package insert, laboratory tests should be checked every 2 weeks for the first 3 months and then monthly thereafter. According to FDA guidelines, cyclosporine should only be used for short-term treatment.

The development of hypertension or decreased renal function does not mean cyclosporine must be discontinued. According to the package insert, if a patient's creatinine increases above baseline by 25% or if the patient's blood pressure is persistently elevated, the dose of cyclosporine can be decreased by 25% to 50% until these values normalize. The dermatologist may need to partner with the primary care physician to help control high blood pressure with antihypertensives. The calcium channel blockers (CCBs) nifedipine (Adalat® CC, Procardia®, Procardia® XL) and isradipine (DynaCirc CR®) are the agents of choice in this situation because they do not alter serum levels of cyclosporine, while verapamil (Calan®, Isoptin® SR) and diltiazem (Cardizem®) are not recommended because they can alter serum levels of cyclosporine. Moreover, some CCBs are thought to protect the kidneys from cyclosporine's nephrotoxic effects. The patient who develops hyperlipidemia may also require the use of lipid-lowering agents.

Other adverse reactions encountered with cyclosporine include GI upset, headache, hypertrichosis, gingival hyperplasia, hyperesthesias and paresthesias. Like those of methotrexate, cyclosporine's side effects are generally reversible and dose-dependent. Cyclosporine is not teratogenic, but it has been associated with low birth weight and premature labor. Physicians should carefully check the manufacturer's prescribing information for a complete list of drug interactions.

Acitretin

Acitretin (Soriatane®) is a synthetic retinoid that normalizes the hyperproliferative state of psoriatic skin by enhancing the maturation and differentiation of keratinocytes. It has a slow onset of action and does not always clear erythema on its own. For these reasons, it is critical to give good patient education regarding what benefit to expect, and in what time frame. However, for nonreproductive patients, it is safe for long-term use with proper supervision and can be used for an unlimited time, provided that no problem develops clinically, radiologically, or with respect to laboratory findings, making it useful for maintenance therapy. It also enhances other modalities of treatment, such as phototherapy, and it is very unusual to have serious drug interactions with other psoriasis treatments (except possibly increasing the risk of hepatotoxicity when used with methotrexate, and therefore the FDA labeled this combination as contraindicated). The combination of retinoids with PUVA or ultraviolet B light (UVB), known as re-PUVA or re-UVB, is very effective and FDA approved. Re-PUVA using a hand and foot machine is one of the best treatments for hand and foot psoriasis. Re-PUVA is also used to transition patients off cyclosporine.

Adverse reactions commonly encountered with acitretin can be uncomfortable for patients. These include significant drying of the mucous membranes, such as the lips and eyes, hair loss, headache, myalgia, decreased night vision, and pyogenic granulomas around the nails. Patients often need to be reassured and provided with symptomatic care. More serious adverse reactions can include an elevation of serum triglycerides and cholesterol, although this is usually easy to control with lipid-lowering agents. Liver function test results can also become abnormally elevated; however, this elevation is often transient, and progression to fibrosis and cirrhosis is almost unknown. A rare side effect of long-term retinoid use is calcification of the ligaments and bony changes in the form of diffuse idiopathic

Table 7-1: Summary of Oral Agents for Psoriasis Treatment

Drug	Dose
Methotrexate (Trexall™)	2.5-5 mg test dose 15-30 mg/wk, divided into 2-3 doses, taken q 8-12 h within 24 h
Cyclosporine (Gengraf®, Neoral®, Sandimmune®)	2.5-4 mg/kg/d divided twice daily
Acitretin (Soriatane®)	10-50 mg once daily

skeletal hyperostosis (DISH) syndrome; however, data are conflicting. Several large, long-term prospective studies failed to show an increased risk of de novo hyperostosis in patients taking acitretin.

Laboratory Tests	Major Toxicities
CBC	Hepatotoxicity
LFTs	Bone marrow suppression
BUN and creatinine	Teratogenicity
Liver biopsy	GI disturbance
Hepatitis screening	

CBC	Nephrotoxicity
LFTs	Hypertension
BUN and creatinine	Hyperlipidemia
Potassium and magnesium	Hypertrichosis
Fasting lipid profile	Hyperesthesia
Hepatitis screening	Paresthesias

CBC	Mucocutaneous xerosis
LFTs	Hyperlipidemia
Fasting lipid profile	Teratogenicity
Pregnancy test	Hepatotoxicity
	Hyperostosis

BUN= blood urea nitrogen; CBC=complete blood count
GI=gastrointestinal; LFT=liver function test

Depression is an adverse reaction allegedly associated with retinoids and is the subject of much controversy. Only isotretinoin (Accutane®) has been linked to depression and suicide, although this association is also controversial.

The extrapolation of this association to other retinoids such as acitretin has not been scientifically substantiated. However, it is sound medicolegal practice to inform the patient of the controversial relationship between depression and retinoids, screen for any mood disorders, and instruct the patient to inform his or her dermatologist about any mood changes. If a mood disturbance occurs, acitretin should be discontinued immediately.

Before initiating therapy, patients must have a baseline CBC, fasting lipid profile, and liver function tests performed. If these evaluations are within normal limits, acitretin can be started at a dose of 25 mg/d. The medication should always be taken with food because this significantly increases its absorption. The dose can be titrated upward as tolerated in increments of 10 mg up to a usual maximum of 50 mg/d. Since acitretin is mostly used for maintenance purposes, 25 mg/d or less, which is considered low-dose, is usually adequate. Laboratory tests should be repeated 2 wk after the initial dose or a dose increase, then in 4 wk, and then again in 8 wk. Monitoring may be as infrequent as once every 3 months for long-term, low-dose (≤25 mg/d) maintenance therapy. Acitretin is known to enhance the efficacy of UVB and PUVA and to decrease the amount of light exposure required to control the disease. When re-PUVA or re-UVB is used, an acitretin dose of 25 mg/d is usually adequate to achieve good enhancement of phototherapy.

Because acitretin is a Category X drug, women should not conceive while on this drug and for a minimum of 3 years after the last dose. This drug should be avoided in women of childbearing potential, especially those who plan on having children in the near future. Those who are of reproductive age and do not plan on having children should be educated about the teratogenic potential of acitretin and instructed to use two effective forms of birth control during therapy and for a minimum of 3 years posttreatment. They should start acitretin on the second or third day after menses has started and be monitored with regular urine pregnancy tests. When choosing oral contraceptives, it is important to know that acitretin may interfere with the effectiveness of the progestin 'minipill.' Men are unaffected and can be reassured that acitretin will not affect their reproductive potential. Because active metabolites can be present in the blood for up to 3 years posttreatment, patients should also be instructed not to donate blood during therapy and for 3 years afterward.

While acitretin has few drug interactions, several are worth noting. Milk can increase its absorption, and vitamin A can increase its toxicity. Taking tetracycline concomitantly has been associated with an increase in the extremely rare incidence of pseudotumor cerebri. Ethanol can increase the half-life of acitretin in the body and should be avoided during and for up to 2 months after treatment, especially in women. Physicians should carefully check the manufacturer's prescribing information for a complete list of drug interactions.

Table 7-1 summarizes available oral agents for psoriasis treatment.

Selected Readings

Callen JP, Kulp-Shorten CL, Wolverton SE: Methotrexate. In: Wolverton SE, ed: *Comprehensive Dermatologic Drug Therapy*. Philadelphia, PA, WB Saunders Co, 2001, pp 147-164.

Goldfarb MT, Ellis CN: Clinical use of etretinate and acitretin. In: Roenigk HH, Maibach HI, eds: *Psoriasis*, 3rd ed. New York, NY, Marcel Dekker, 1998, pp 663-670.

Koo JY, Gambla C, Lee J: Cyclosporin for the treatment of psoriasis. In: Roenigk HH, Maibach HI, eds: *Psoriasis*, 3rd ed. New York, NY, Marcel Dekker, 1998, pp 641-658.

Koo JY, Lee CS, Maloney JE: Cyclosporine and related drugs. In: Wolverton SE, ed: *Comprehensive Dermatologic Drug Therapy*. Philadelphia, PA, WB Saunders Co, 2001, pp 205-229.

Lebwohl MG, Feldman SR, Koo JY, et al: *Psoriasis: Treatment Options and Patient Management*. National Psoriasis Foundation, 2002, pp 45-72.

Roenigk HH, Maibach HI: Methotrexate. In: Roenigk HH, Maibach HI, eds: *Psoriasis*, 3rd ed. New York, NY, Marcel Dekker, 1998, pp 609-630.

Smith C, Barker J, Menter MA: *Psoriasis*. Oxford, England, Health Press, 2002, pp 51-56.

Wright S, Gemzik B: Hydroxyurea. In: Roenigk HH, Maibach HI, eds: *Psoriasis*, 3rd ed. New York, NY, Marcel Dekker, 1998, pp 631-636.

Chapter 8

Goeckerman Therapy

Goeckerman therapy is one of the oldest regimens for treating psoriasis. Despite the excitement generated by newer oral agents and injectable biologics, inpatient therapy remains one of the fastest, safest, and most effective treatments for moderate-to-severe psoriasis. Data from the University of California San Francisco Psoriasis Treatment Center show that PASI 75 (≥75% improvement in the Psoriasis Area Severity Index [PASI]) at 3 months with Goeckerman therapy is 100%. Additionally, among published data on average remission times with various psoriasis therapies, Goeckerman therapy offers the longest known remission time (Figures 8-1 and 8-2, see color insert). Moreover, the data from the Mayo Clinic suggest that Goeckerman therapy is effective in most patients who failed biologic agents. A review of our Goeckerman data at UCSF Psoriasis Treatment Center for the past 5 years is in accord with the conclusion of the Mayo Clinic report.

Traditionally, Goeckerman therapy took place in an inpatient setting. It was a 24-hour-per-day treatment course until patients were discharged. Because of problems with reimbursement under managed care, and because of the inconvenience to patients, this course has become a daycare procedure in most facilities today. Patients are treated 8 hours/day, 5 days/week, until their disease clears, which usually takes 20 to 30 treatment days. Patients typically begin the day with ultraviolet B (UVB) phototherapy. Following light treatment, crude coal tar in concentrations up to 10% (often with salicylic acid or lactic acid) is applied to the entire body, including normal skin.

Intertriginous areas are avoided unless they contain psoriasis. Patients are then wrapped with plastic wrap for occlusive purposes, and dressed in old pajamas or scrubs. After they are fully dressed, their scalp is treated with 20% liquor carbonis detergens (LCD) (see description in Chapter 5) and occluded with a shower cap. Patients can then relax until the afternoon. To remove the tar, they use mineral oil and routine showering. Finally, brown tar (20% LCD in Aquaphor®) is applied before going home and again at bedtime. The most critical detail contributing to the high efficacy of Goeckerman therapy is the use of black crude coal tar rather than refined or diluted tar preparations, which are typically brown or gold in appearance (Figure 8-3, see color insert).

In some patients, psoriasis clears in as little as 2 weeks. More severely affected patients require longer treatments. For these patients, additional therapies can be combined with Goeckerman therapy. Modern use of Goeckerman therapy often includes the original ingredients of UVB phototherapy and black tar supplemented with other modalities, including anthralin, salicylic acid, lactic acid, vitamin D analogues (Dovonex®, Vectical®), and tazarotene (Tazorac®). Bath-psoralen plus ultraviolet A (PUVA) phototherapy can be added for resistant cases or resistant anatomic locations. Extremely treatment-resistant patients who are receiving UVB and PUVA phototherapy sequentially, on the same day, should receive UVB first, before the application of psoralen, to avoid inadvertent exposure to contaminating UVA wavelengths while receiving UVB phototherapy.

In the past, Goeckerman therapy was widely practiced in the United States as the 'gold standard' for psoriasis. With the advent of managed care, there are only a few places equipped to perform traditional Goeckerman therapy. Overseas, this therapy remains an essential treatment option, especially for severe disease.

Selected Readings

Horwitz S: Ultraviolet therapy with coal tars. In: Lowe NJ, ed: *Practical Psoriasis Therapy*, 2nd ed. St. Louis, MO, Mosby-Year Book, 1993, pp 95-113.

Koo J, Lebwohl M: Duration of remission of psoriasis therapies. *J Am Acad Dermatol* 1999;41:51-59.

Koo JY, Lebwohl MG, Lee CS, eds: *Mild-to-Moderate Psoriasis*. Informa Healthcare USA, Inc, New York, NY, 2006.

Lee E, Koo J: Modern modified 'ultra' Goeckerman therapy: a PASI assessment of a very effective therapy for psoriasis resistant to both prebiologic and biologic therapies. *J Dermatolog Treat* 2005; 16:102-107.

Serrao R, Davis M: Goeckerman treatment for remission of psoriasis refractory to biologic therapy. *J Am Acad Dermatol* 2009;60: 348-349.

Chapter 9

Combination, Rotational, and Sequential Therapies

Optimizing therapy for patients with psoriasis that is resistant to usual therapies requires the use of creative therapeutic strategies, such as combination, rotational, and sequential therapies, which involves balancing many factors, including safety, efficacy, onset of action, and duration of response.

Using two agents that work through different mechanisms of action can maximize therapeutic results by merging the strengths and minimizing the weaknesses of each. For example, an agent with a rapid onset of action but with a less favorable side-effect profile can be used in sequence with a slower-acting, less toxic agent. The drug used for its speed of action can then be tapered, and the patient maintained on the slower but safer agent. Cyclosporine (Gengraf®, Neoral®) works quickly and effectively, but is not suitable for long-term use because of its nephrotoxic potential. Acitretin (Soriatane®) is safer to use for extended periods but has a slow onset of action. Using both agents in sequence combines the benefits of rapid clearance with safe maintenance. This particular 'rabbit to turtle' strategy has been devised by the author (Dr. J. Koo), who coined the term *sequential therapy*. Another benefit of using multiple agents is that patients can usually achieve the same response on doses of agents used in combination that are much lower than those required when each is used as a monotherapy. A good example of this phenomenon is the use of retinoids with phototherapy, which is approved by the Food and Drug

Administration (FDA). Doses of acitretin and cumulative exposure to ultraviolet B (UVB) or psoralen plus ultraviolet A (PUVA) can be reduced when acitretin and phototherapy are used together. Certain combinations are to be avoided, particularly cyclosporine and phototherapy, because of the increased risk of skin cancer with long-term use, especially in fair-skinned Caucasian patients.

Rotational Therapy

Rotational therapy minimizes cumulative toxicity by switching between agents with differing toxicity profiles. Many systemic agents have side effects that are dose-dependent and reversible upon discontinuation of the drug. Therapies such as cyclosporine cannot be used for an extended period on an uninterrupted basis. By switching from one therapeutic regimen to another, the patient is given a 'holiday' from one particular treatment.

Sequential Therapy

Sequential therapy is a commonly employed strategy in which agents are used in a deliberate sequence to maximize the initial speed of improvement while minimizing long-term toxicity. The three phases of sequential therapy are step 1, the clearing phase; step 2, the transition phase; and step 3, the maintenance phase (Table 9-1).

The classic example of topical sequential therapy involves a vitamin D analogue (Dovonex®, Vectical®) and a class I super-potent topical steroid. Super-potent topical cortico-steroids are more efficacious and work more rapidly than a vitamin D analogue. However, long-term use can result in skin atrophy and adrenal suppression. A vitamin D analogue is effective over time and safe to use long term, but is slower to act and associated with irritation. Using both medications sequentially optimizes the rate and degree of clearance by combining their strengths and allowing them to coun-teract individual weaknesses. When used simultaneously but applied separately, there is a synergistic enhancement

Table 9-1: Sequential Therapy

Topical Sequential Therapy

Step 1	Step 2
Vitamin D analogue (Dovonex®, Vectical®) + super-potent topical steroid twice daily ~2 weeks to 1 month	Vitamin D analogue twice daily on weekdays Vitamin D analogue + super-potent topical steroid twice daily on weekends ~1 month

Repeatable Sequential Therapy

Step 1	Step 2
Clobetasol (Clobex®) spray twice daily for 1 month	Calcitriol (Vectical®) ointment twice daily for 1 month or longer

Systemic Sequential Therapy

Step 1	Step 2
Cyclosporine ~1 month	Transition to acitretin

PUVA=psoralen plus ultraviolet A; UVB=ultraviolet B;
BSA=body surface area

of efficacy, and improvement can be more rapid than when either agent is used alone. The presence of a steroid decreases the risk of vitamin D analogue irritation, while maintenance with a vitamin D analogue eliminates the risk of skin atrophy and adrenal suppression that is associated with long-term

Step 3

Vitamin D analogue twice daily.
Indefinitely or until clearance[*]

Step 3

This sequence is repeatable once
psoriasis recurs to involve ≥3% BSA.

Step 3

Add UVB or PUVA. Maintain on
retinoids with UVB (re-UVB) or
retinoids with PUVA (re-PUVA).
Indefinitely or until clearance[*]

[*]Depends on the natural history of psoriasis for the particular
patient being treated.

steroid use. The gradual transition off steroids prevents the
rebound that can occur after abrupt discontinuation.

Step 1 consists of using both agents, twice daily. If the
patient is compliant with this regimen, clearance often occurs in approximately 1 month. During the transition phase,

a gradual tapering of the steroid takes place. A vitamin D analogue alone is used twice daily on weekdays, while the combination is used twice daily on weekends to 'pulse' the patient with steroids. The patient usually continues step 2 for approximately 1 month, but some resistant cases may require steroid pulse therapy longer (ie, weekday/weekend regimen). If periodically supervised, patients can be safely maintained on step 2 long term, since it would be extremely unusual for a patient to develop adrenal suppression or skin atrophy when using topical steroids only 2 days/week. Most patients should begin step 3 as soon as possible, which consists of maintenance with a vitamin D analogue alone, twice daily. If relapse occurs, the patient can be moved back to step 2 or step 1 and then switched to step 3 as control of the disease is attained again. This original, sequential therapy strategy has been widely practiced worldwide with good effect. However, the main drawback is that the regimen is rather complicated; therefore, the compliance, especially for the later steps, becomes more difficult once the patient is out of the acute misery and the motivation for skin therapy diminishes.

The same 'rabbit-to-turtle' model of sequential therapy can be used with clobetasol spray and calcitriol ointment. This strategy involves alternating monthly between monotherapy with clobetasol spray twice daily and monotherapy with calcitriol ointment twice daily (Figure 9-1). With 4 weeks of a 'steroid holiday' between treatment cycles, it is safe and, with regards to timeline, within FDA labeling to restart clobetasol spray for another a 1-month duration, thereby unleashing the most powerful intervention before psoriasis has the chance to deteriorate. According to the package insert, this strategy uses each treatment one at a time as monotherapy with treatment times limited to on-label instructions. By repeating this proposed regimen, the previously mentioned data suggest that our specialty now has a strategy to attain our age-old goal for optimally controlling psoriasis—a double challenge of attaining

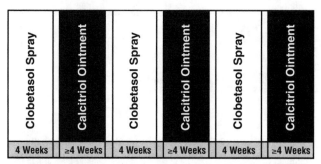

Figure 9-1: Sequential therapy with alternating regimens of pharmacologic treatment. To be in line with FDA labeling, clobetasol spray can be restarted after a "steroid holiday" once psoriasis involves ≥3% BSA.

(1) a quick, effective, and very reliable initial control, and (2) safely maintaining that control *without* allowing clinical deterioration.

Selected Readings

Emer J, Lebwohl MG: Combination, rotational, and sequential therapies. In: Koo JYM, Lee CS, Lebwohl MG, et al, eds. *Moderate to Severe Psoriasis*. New York, Informa Healthcare USA, 2009, pp 193-218.

Koo JY: Sequential therapy of psoriasis. Introducing a new therapeutic paradigm for better clinical results. *J Am Acad Dermatol* 1999;41:S25-S28.

Koo J: How and why to employ sequential therapy for psoriasis. *Skin Aging* 2000;(suppl):16-21.

Koo J: Systemic sequential therapy of psoriasis: a new paradigm for improved therapeutic results. *J Am Acad Dermatol* 1999;41 (3 pt 2):S25-S28.

Lebwohl MG: Combination, rotational, and sequential therapy. In: Weinstein GD, Gottlieb AB, eds: *Therapy of Moderate-to-Severe Psoriasis*, 2nd ed. New York, NY, Marcel Dekker, 2003, pp 179-196.

Lebwohl MG, Feldman SR, Koo JY, et al: *Psoriasis: Treatment Options and Patient Management*. Portland, OR, National Psoriasis Foundation, 2002, pp 21-26.

Chapter 10

The Biologic Agents

Biologic agents can be thought of as the strategic 'smart bombs' of the systemic immunomodulators. They are custom made and designed to interact with specific targets within the immune system, minimizing the collateral organ damage seen with the use of generalized immunomodulators, such as cyclosporine (Gengraf®, Neoral®, Sandimmune®) and methotrexate (Trexall™). The biologics are bioengineered proteins that bind to receptor sites on T cells or the cytokines they produce, blocking T-cell activation, killing T cells, blocking T-cell migration, or interfering with the action of cytokines and thereby inhibiting the inflammatory cascade.

Because the biologics are immunomodulators, there is concern about their potential to make patients more susceptible to infection or malignancy. The *Physician's Desk Reference®* and individual package inserts contain warnings about the possible increased risk of developing these adverse events. Indeed, rare cases of serious infection and malignancy have been reported with the use of each drug described in this chapter. However, not every biologic agent has shown convincing evidence of causing or increasing these risks.

A summary of biologic agents for psoriasis is presented in Table 10-1.

Adalimumab

Adalimumab (Humira®) is a human monoclonal antibody that specifically blocks the proinflammatory cytokine tumor necrosis factor-α (TNF-α). In 2002, the US Food and Drug Administration (FDA) approved adalimumab for the treatment of rheumatoid arthritis, and subsequently approved the drug for the treatment of ankylosing spondylitis, psoriatic arthritis, Crohn's disease, and juvenile arthritis. In January 2008, the FDA approved adalimumab for the treatment of moderate to severe chronic plaque psoriasis in patients who are candidates for systemic therapy or phototherapy, and when other systemic therapies are medically less appropriate. Thus far, more than 460,000 patients worldwide have been treated with adalimumab for its various indications.

The recommended dose of adalimumab for adult patients with plaque psoriasis is an initial dose of 80 mg followed by a 40-mg dose every other week, starting 1 week after the initial dose. The patient may self-inject adalimumab using either the pen or a prefilled syringe, after he or she has been properly trained by medical personnel in subcutaneous injection technique.

Adalimumab's approval for the treatment of psoriasis was based on multiple clinical studies in which 1,696 patients were treated, with some patients treated for >2 years. The Randomized Controlled Evaluation of Adalimumab Every Other Week Dosing in Moderate to Severe Psoriasis trial (REVEAL) lasted 52 weeks with 1,212 patients enrolled who were treated with either adalimumab 40 mg every other week (starting 1 week after an 80-mg loading dose) or with placebo during the first part of the study. Among adalimumab-treated patients, 71% achieved a Psoriasis Area and Severity Index (PASI) 75 response by week 16 vs 7% in placebo. Later in the study, subjects treated with adalimumab who maintained a PASI 75 response at week 33 were rerandomized to either continue treatment or switched to placebo. After 52 weeks of treatment, more patients on adalimumab (79%) maintained efficacy compared to patients rerandomized to placebo. However, 43% of these placebo patients still maintained a PASI 75 response without any treatment for 19 weeks.

(continued on page 82)

Table 10-1: Summary of Biologic Agents Currently Approved by the FDA for Psoriasis

Drug	Dosing	Laboratory Tests, per FDA	Warnings/ Precautions
Adalimumab (Humira®)	80 mg SC initial dose, followed by 40 mg every other week, starting 1 wk after initial dose	Screening with PPD or QuantiFERON®-TB Gold is required. If positive, chest x-ray and pretreatment with anti-TB agent(s) are required. PPD and QuantiFERON®-TB Gold should be tested periodically during treatment. Optional monitoring includes baseline and/or periodic hepatitis profile, liver function tests, and CBC	Most common is injection site reaction. Small risk for infections (URI, bronchitis, UTI). Rare risk of serious and opportunistic infections; reactivation of tuberculosis; reactivation of hepatitis B virus in chronic carriers; invasive fungal infections (such as histoplasmosis)*

URI=upper respiratory infections; UTI=urinary tract infections

*Lymphoma and other malignancies, some fatal, have been reported in children and adolescent patients treated with TNF blockers.

Current Indications

Moderate to severe chronic plaque psoriasis

Psoriatic arthritis

Rheumatoid arthritis

Ankylosing spondylitis

Juvenile idiopathic arthritis

Crohn's disease

Efficacy Data

Following 16 wk of treatment at a dose of 40 mg every other week after an 80-mg initial dose, 71% of patients achieved ≥75% improvement in PASI score, or 45% achieved 90% clearance, while 62% of patients had a PGA score of clear or minimal

CBC=complete blood count; PASI=Psoriasis Area and Severity Index: a clinical assessment performed by physicians, which rates the overall severity of psoriasis based on erythema, plaque thickness, scaling, and affected body surface area (BSA); PGA=physician global assessment; PPD=purified protein derivative; SC=subcutaneously; TB=tuberculosis

(continued on next page)

Table 10-1: Summary of Biologic Agents Currently Approved by the FDA for Psoriasis (continued)

Drug	Dosing	Laboratory Tests, per FDA	Warnings/ Precautions
Alefacept (Amevive®)	15 mg IM, office	CD4 counts every other week (dosing held for CD4 less than 250). Consider pre-treatment HIV test.	Small risk for infections (URI, bronchitis, UTI) and decreased T-lymphocyte levels (CD4 and CD8). Rare risk of serious and opportunistic infections; malignancies including nonmelanoma skin cancers; and hypersensitivity reactions such as angioedema or urticaria, have been reported.

Current Indications

Moderate to severe chronic plaque psoriasis

Efficacy Data

At week 14 (ie, 2 weeks after the last IM injection), 21% achieved ≥75% improvement in PASI and 14% of patients had a PGA score of clear or almost clear. The peak average PASI improvement is seen at week 18 (ie, 6 wk after the last IM injection).

10

IM=intramuscular; PASI=Psoriasis Area and Severity Index: a clinical assessment performed by physicians, which rates the overall severity of psoriasis based on erythema, plaque thickness, scaling, and affected body surface area (BSA); PGA=physician global assessment

(continued on next page)

Table 10-1: Summary of Biologic Agents Currently Approved by the FDA for Psoriasis (continued)

Drug	Dosing	Laboratory Tests, per FDA	Warnings/Precautions
Etanercept (Enbrel®)	50 mg SC twice weekly for the first 3 months. After first 3 months, 50 mg once weekly.	Screening with PPD or QuantiFERON®-TB Gold is required. If positive, chest x-ray and pretreatment with anti-TB agent(s) are required. PPD and QuantiFERON®-TB Gold should be tested periodically during treatment. Optional monitoring includes baseline and/or periodic hepatitis profile, liver function tests, and CBC.	Small risk for infections (URI, bronchitis, UTI). Rare risk of serious and opportunistic infections; reactivation of TB; reactivation of hepatitis B virus in chronic carriers; invasive fungal infections (such as histoplasmosis); demyelinating disease, exacerbation or new onset; or exacerbation of congestive heart failure*

*Lymphoma and other malignancies, some fatal, have been reported in children and adolescent patients treated with TNF blockers.

Current Indications

Psoriatic arthritis

Rheumatoid arthritis

Ankylosing spondylitis

Chronic moderate to severe plaque psoriasis

Polyarticular juvenile idiopathic arthritis

Efficacy Data

PASI ≥75% in about 49% of patients in 12 wk at 50 mg SC twice weekly

47% of patients had a PGA score of clear or minimal

CBC=complete blood count; PASI=Psoriasis Area and Severity Index: a clinical assessment performed by physicians, which rates the overall severity of psoriasis based on erythema, plaque thickness, scaling, and affected body surface area (BSA); PGA=physician global assessment; PPD=purified protein derivative; SC=subcutaneously; TB=tuberculosis

(continued on next page)

Table 10-1: Summary of Biologic Agents Currently Approved by the FDA for Psoriasis (continued)

Drug	Dosing	Laboratory Tests, per FDA	Warnings/ Precautions
Infliximab (Remicade®)	Approved IV dose is 5 mg/kg body weight at 0, 2, 6 weeks, then every 8 wk	Screening with PPD or QuantiFERON®-TB Gold is required. If positive, chest x-ray and pre-treatment with anti-TB agent(s) are required. PPD and QuantiFERON®-TB Gold should be tested periodically during treatment. Baseline and/or periodic hepatic profile and liver function tests are also highly recommended. Optional monitoring includes CBC	Small risk for infections (URI, bronchitis, UTI). Rare risk of serious and opportunistic infections; reactivation of TB; reactivation of hepatitis B virus in chronic carriers; invasive fungal infections (such as histoplasmosis); demyelinating disease, exacerbation or new onset; malignancies including hepatosplenic T-cell lymphoma; hepatotoxicity; hypersensitivity reactions including anaphylaxis or serum sickness; or exacerbation of congestive heart failure

Current Indications

Adult and pediatric Crohn's disease

Chronic severe plaque psoriasis

Psoriatic arthritis

Ankylosing spondylitis

Ulcerative colitis

Rheumatoid arthritis

Efficacy Data

PASI ≥75% achieved by about 80% of patients in about 10-12 wk at 5 mg/kg dosing

80% also had a PGA score of clear or minimal

CBC=complete blood count; IV=intravenous; PASI=Psoriasis Area and Severity Index: a clinical assessment performed by physicians, which rates the overall severity of psoriasis based on erythema, plaque thickness, scaling, and affected body surface area (BSA); PGA=physician global assessment; PPD=purified protein derivative; TB=tuberculosis

(continued on next page)

Table 10-1: Summary of Biologic Agents Currently Approved by the FDA for Psoriasis (continued)

Drug	Dosing	Laboratory Tests, per FDA	Warnings/ Precautions
Ustekinumab (Stelara®)	Patients ≤100 kg, 45 mg SC at weeks 0, 4, and then every 12 wk Patients >100 kg, 90 mg SC at weeks 0, 4, and then every 12 wk	Screening with PPD or QuantiFERON®-TB Gold is required. If positive, chest x-ray and pretreatment with anti-TB agent(s) are required. PPD and QuantiFERON®-TB Gold should be tested periodically during treatment. Optional monitoring includes baseline and/or periodic hepatitis profile, liver function tests, and CBC	Small risk for infections (URI, bronchitis, UTI). Rare risk of serious bacterial, viral, and fungal infections; reactivation of TB; and reversible posterior leukoencephalopathy syndrome

Current Indications

Moderate to severe plaque type psoriasis

Efficacy Data

In one trial, at week 12, 67.1% of patients on 45-mg dose and 66.7% on 90-mg dose achieved PASI 75. In another trial, PASI 75 at 12 wk was seen in 66.4% and 75.7% in the 45-mg and 90-mg groups, respectively.

In study 1, 59% of patients on 45-mg dose and 61% of patients on 90-mg dose had a PGA of clear or minimal.

In study 2, 68% of patients on 45-mg dose and 73% of patients on 90-mg dose had a PGA of clear or minimal.

10

CBC=complete blood count; PASI=Psoriasis Area and Severity Index: a clinical assessment performed by physicians, which rates the overall severity of psoriasis based on erythema, plaque thickness, scaling, and affected body surface area (BSA); PGA=physician global assessment; PPD=purified protein derivative; SC=subcutaneously; TB=tuberculosis

None of the patients who were rerandomized to the placebo arm at week 33 of the study experienced an aggressive recurrence of their psoriasis, or rebound. During the REVEAL trial, 8.4% of adalimumab-treated patients developed antibodies to adalimumab, with no apparent relationship between the development of antibodies and loss of adequate response.

Adalimumab is also approved for the treatment of psoriatic arthritis, demonstrating symptom relief and radiographic inhibition of joint damage that could be erosive and destructive. The most common adverse reactions seen in clinical studies were mild and included injection site reactions and mild infections. The most serious adverse reactions seen were serious infections, neurologic reactions, and malignancies.

In the placebo-controlled rheumatoid arthritis trials, the rate of serious infection was 1 per patient year in the patients treated with adalimumab vs 0.9 per patient year in the placebo-treated patients. The infections consisted primarily of upper respiratory tract infections, bronchitis, and urinary tract infections. Most patients continued treatment after the infection resolved. The incidence of serious infections for RA patients was 0.04 per patient year in adalimumab-treated RA patients and 0.02 per patient year in placebo-treated patients. Serious infections observed included pneumonia, septic arthritis, prosthetic and postsurgical infections, erysipelas, cellulitis, diverticulitis, and pyleonephritis.

Patients should be monitored closely for serious infections. Serious and potentially fatal infections, including opportunistic infections and invasive fungal infections such as *Histoplasma*, *Aspergillus*, and *Nocardia* infections, have been reported in patients receiving TNF-α antagonists, including adalimumab. The FDA recommends that adalimumab should be used with caution in patients who have previously or are residing in an area where histoplasmosis is endemic.

In completed and ongoing clinical studies that include more than 13,000 patients, the average rate of tuberculosis

(TB) is approximately 0.26 per 100 patient years. Most of the cases of TB occurred within the first 8 months after initiation of therapy and may reflect recrudescence of latent disease. The risk of reactivation of latent TB has made prescreening the standard of care for all TNF-α antagonists. When tuberculin skin testing is performed for latent TB infection, an induration size of ≥5 mm should be considered positive. For patients who have been vaccinated previously with Bacille Calmette-Guerin (BCG), the QuantiFERON®-TB Gold test is available. If latent infection is diagnosed, appropriate treatment should be started prior to starting TNF-α antagonist therapy, in accordance with the current Centers for Disease Control and Prevention (CDC) guidelines. If latent infection is diagnosed, a chest x-ray should also be performed to rule out active TB. If necessary, consultation should occur with a physician who has expertise in the treatment of TB.

Patients should also be counseled about the risk of lymphoma and other malignancies while receiving adalimumab. The authors recommend that adalimumab should be avoided in patients with malignancy or history of malignancy. Adalimumab should be promptly discontinued in patients who develop malignancy while on therapy. Additionally, while studies evaluating adalimumab for treatment of psoriasis did not report any cases of demyelinating disease, national guidelines suggest that adalimumab should not be used in patients with demyelinating diseases or in those with first-degree relatives with multiple sclerosis. Patients should also be advised to seek immediate medical attention if they experience any symptoms of severe allergic reactions. Latex-sensitive patients need to be advised that the needle cap of the prefilled syringe contains latex. In addition, patients should be advised to report any signs of new or worsening medical conditions, such as heart disease, neurologic disease, or autoimmune disorders, and should report any symptoms suggestive of cytopenia, including bruising, bleeding, or persistent fever.

Alefacept

Alefacept (Amevive®) is a fusion protein combining a portion of human immunoglobulin (IgG) and the binding site of lymphocyte function-associated antigen-3 (LFA-3). It binds to CD2, the partner molecule of LFA-3 located on the surface of T cells. This drug also binds to the surface proteins of accessory cells, including natural killer cells and macrophages. Alefacept inhibits T-cell activation and proliferation and also induces T-cell apoptosis. Because it depletes a subset of CD4 T cells, the absolute CD4 count may decline and must be monitored during treatment.

Alefacept is administered via intramuscular (IM) injection. A dosing course consists of 12 weekly administrations of 15 mg IM. Absolute CD4 counts must be performed every other week during treatment, and the dose must be held if the CD4 count drops below 250 cells/mm^3. Patients can have repeated courses of alefacept, as long as their CD4 counts are within normal range and at least 12 weeks have elapsed between courses.

In an international, randomized, double-blind, placebo-controlled trial, Lebwohl et al evaluated the efficacy and tolerability of alefacept in 507 patients with chronic plaque psoriasis. Patients were given placebo, alefacept 10 mg, or alefacept 15 mg once a week for a total of 12 weeks. This study found that IM alefacept was well tolerated and effective, with 24% of the patients in the 15-mg group, 22% of patients in the 10-mg group, and 8% of the patients in the placebo group assessed as being clear or almost clear of psoriasis at 12-week follow-up. Mean PASI score reductions were 46% in the 15-mg group, 41% in the 10-mg group, and 25% in the placebo group at 6 weeks post-dosing.

In another double-blind, placebo-controlled, parallel-group study by Ellis et al, patients with chronic plaque psoriasis were given alefacept 0.025 mg/kg body weight, 0.075 mg/kg body weight, 0.150 mg/kg body weight, or placebo. This study used intravenous (IV) dosing, which was subsequently removed from the US market. The patients received one infusion/week for 12 wk. Twelve wk after treatment, 47%, 63%, and 42% of the three alefacept-treatment groups, respectively, had at least a 50% reduction in their baseline PASI scores. Of the patients who had received alefacept, 24% were clear or almost clear of psoriasis, compared with 5% of those patients who had received placebo.

While onset of action is slow, improvement with alefacept progresses over time, and patients typically continue to exhibit improvement even after the last dose of a course. Practitioners and patients should be realistic about how slowly they will see clinical benefit, which typically peaks at week 18 (ie, 6 wk after the last dose of a 12-wk course). A major benefit of alefacept is that it is a remittive therapy, and the median duration of response maintaining at least 50% improvement is 7 to 8 months among patients who achieve ≥75% improvement in PASI any time during the 3-month treatment (injection) period. With IM alefacept, 33% of patients achieve this level of improvement within the 6-month period. Alefacept is well tolerated, with no evidence of major organ toxicity or rebound after treatment has been completed. For psoriasis, alefacept was the first biologic to be approved and therefore has the longest postmarketing database of all biologics used for psoriasis.

Because of its tolerability and favorable side-effect profile, alefacept may be well suited for long-term, intermittent use. It can also be a valuable agent for a patient who develops side effects from traditional systemic agents or who does not want to assume the potential risks associated with them. Alefacept is an especially useful option for a patient who has comorbidities for which medications such as methotrexate, cyclosporine, or anti-TNF biologic agents are absolutely or relatively contraindicated.

Etanercept

Etanercept (Enbrel®) is a fusion protein consisting of two TNF receptors fused to the Fc portion of human immunoglobulin G (IgG) antibody. This construct creates an exogenous TNF receptor and prevents excess TNF from binding to cell-bound receptors. Etanercept binds to both TNF-α and TNF-β. The end result is a reduction of active TNF and mitigation of diseases, such as rheumatoid arthritis and psoriasis, which are mediated by the effects of TNF.

Etanercept has been used in more than 500,000 patients and is approved by the FDA for the treatment of psoriasis, psoriatic arthritis, ankylosing spondylitis, and juvenile idiopathic and adult rheumatoid arthritis. Etanercept has been shown to be effective as monotherapy for moderate to severe plaque psoriasis. One randomized, controlled trial evaluated 672 patients who received either placebo, etanercept 25 mg once weekly, etanercept 25 mg twice weekly, or etanercept 50 mg twice weekly for 3 months. At 12 weeks, 14% of patients achieved PASI 75 in the 25-mg per week group, 32% in the 25-mg twice-a-week group, and 47% in the 50-mg twice-a-week group versus 7% in the placebo group. After 3 months, patients continued on blinded treatment for an additional 3 months, at which time patients originally randomized to placebo began treatment with blinded etanercept at 25 mg twice a week. After 24 wk, 21% of patients achieved PASI 75 in the 25-mg per week group, 41% in the 25-mg twice-a-week group, and 54% in the 50-mg twice-a-week group compared to 33% in the placebo-to-etanercept group. Another study evaluated 611 patients who received placebo or etanercept at doses of 25 mg or 50 mg twice weekly for 3 months. At 12 wk, 32% of patients in the 25-mg twice-a-week group achieved PASI 75 versus 46% in the 50-mg twice-a-week group and only 3% in the placebo group.

Infections, including viral, bacterial, and fungal infections, have been observed in clinical trials. In the controlled portions of all the pivotal trials, the types and severity of infection were similar between etanercept and the respective control group. Infections consisted primarily of upper respiratory tract infections, sinusitis, and influenza. The rates of serious infections were also similar—0.8% in placebo vs 1.4% in etanercept. In clinical trials in psoriasis, serious infections experienced by patients included pneumonia, cellulitis, gastroenteritis, abscess, and osteomyelitis. The rate of serious infections was not increased in open-label extension trials and was similar to that in etanercept-treated and placebo-treated patients from controlled clinical trials.

In 66 global clinical trials of 17,505 patients, TB was observed in approximately 0.02% of patients. Data from clinical trials and preclinical studies suggest that the risk of reactivation of latent TB infection is lower than with TNF-blocking monoclonal antibodies. Nonetheless, postmarketing cases of TB reactivation have been reported for TNF blockers, including etanercept. Therefore, patients must be evaluated for TB risk factors and tested for latent infection with PPD and/or QuantiFERON®-TB Gold testing prior to initiating etanercept and periodically during therapy. Anti-tuberculosis therapy should also be strongly considered before initiation of etanercept in patients with a history of latent or active TB in whom an adequate course of treatment cannot be confirmed.

Other serious adverse events have also been described. Treatment with TNF blocking agents, including etanercept, has been associated with rare (<0.1%) cases of new onset or exacerbation of CNS demyelinating disorders. Physicians should exercise caution in considering the use of etanercept in patients with preexisting or recent onset CNS demyelinating disorders. Many patients may also express concerns about malignancies. Among 1,245 adult psoriasis patients treated with etanercept in controlled clinical trials, representing approximately 283 patient years of therapy, the observed rate of nonmelanoma skin cancer (NMSC) was 3.54 cases per 100 patient years vs 1.28 cases per 100 patient years among 720 control-treated patients representing 156 patient years. Therefore, periodic skin examinations should be considered for all patients. However, among 4,410 adult psoriasis patients treated with etanercept in clinical trials up to 36 months, the observed rate of lymphoma was 0.05 cases per 100 patient years, which is comparable to the rate in the general population. For malignancies, other than lymphoma and NMSC, there was no difference in exposure adjusted rates between the etanercept and control arms.

Etanercept, for the treatment of psoriasis, has been approved for induction dosing of 50 mg subcutaneously twice a week for the first 3 months. After this 3-month induction phase, the dose of etanercept must be decreased to 50 mg once a week or 25 mg twice a week for maintenance regimen. However, some patients may deteriorate with regard to their psoriasis when the dose is decreased (as specified by the FDA). Patients who are overweight or obese are at greater risk for deterioration in their psoriasis status as compared with patients who are not overweight.

Infliximab

Infliximab (Remicade®) is a monoclonal antibody that targets TNF and is administered intravenously. An initial infusion is given, followed by repeat administrations 2 and 6 weeks later. Patients can then be maintained with an infusion every several months. Infliximab is now indicated for the treatment of rheumatoid arthritis and Crohn's disease, ankylosing spondylitis, ulcerative colitis, psoriatic arthritis, and adults with chronic, severe plaque psoriasis who are candidates for systemic therapy or when other systemic therapies are inappropriate.

In September 2006, infliximab was approved for the treatment of psoriasis. Commonly reported side effects include nonspecific symptoms, such as headache and diarrhea. Screening for tuberculosis before starting therapy is particularly important because infliximab has been associated with rare incidents of reactivation of tuberculosis in patients with latent infection. A few cases of sepsis and opportunistic infections such as histoplasmosis have been reported with use of this agent. In patients with congestive heart failure, infliximab should be avoided. A significant percentage of patients who take infliximab develop antibodies against the nonhuman portion of the drug.

In studies of patients with moderate-to-severe psoriasis, infliximab has been shown to provide a rapid response as well as a high probability of attaining 75% or better improvement in PASI (PASI 75). Two phase III trials have been conducted. In the Express 1 trial (n=378), 80% of patients on 5 mg/kg induction dose achieved PASI 75 by week 10. However, by week 50 only 61% of patients getting 5 mg/kg every 8 wk maintained a PASI 75 response. In the Express 2 trial (n=835), 76% of patients achieved PASI 75 with the 5-mg/kg induction dose at week 10. Consult the latest *Physician's Desk Reference*® for the full prescribing information on infliximab because several possible serious side effects ranging from rare cases of hepatotoxicity to hepatic cancers have been reported.

Ustekinumab

Ustekinumab (Stelara®) is a human IgG1-kappa monoclonal antibody antagonist of the p40 subunit of IL-12 and IL-23. Ustekinumab is indicated for psoriasis through targeted antagonism of these two inflammatory cytokines. Ustekinumab was FDA approved in September 2009 for treatment of patients 18 years of age and older with moderate-to-severe plaque-type psoriasis who are eligible for phototherapy or systemic therapy.

Two large, phase III clinical trials were conducted to determine the efficacy and safety of ustekinumab. The first trial, PHOENIX 1, was a multicenter, parallel, double-blind, placebo-controlled study of 766 psoriasis patients who were randomly assigned to receive ustekinumab 45 mg, or 90 mg at weeks 0, 4, and every 12 weeks thereafter, or placebo at weeks 0 and 4 with crossover to ustekinumab treatment at week 12. A PASI 75 response at week 12 was achieved by 171 (67.1%) patients in the 45-mg ustekinumab group, by 170 (66.4%) patients in the 90-mg group, and by 8 (3.1%) patients in the placebo group. The second trial, PHOENIX 2, was a multicenter, double-blind, placebo-controlled study of 1,230 psoriasis patients who were randomly assigned to receive ustekinumab 45 mg or 90 mg or placebo at weeks 0, 4, and every 12 weeks thereafter. A PASI 75 response at week 12 was achieved by 273 (66.7%) patients in the 45-mg ustekinumab group, by 311 (75.7%) patients in the 90-mg group, and by 15 (3.7%) patients in the placebo group.

The most common adverse reactions noted in clinical trials included nasopharyngitis, upper respiratory tract infection, and headache. In the controlled periods of the clinical trials, 27% of patients treated with ustekinumab reported infections compared with 24% of placebo-treated patients. Serious infections occurred in 0.3% of patients treated with ustekinumab vs 0.4% treated with placebo. In the controlled and noncontrolled portions of the psoriasis clinical trials, 0.4% of ustekinumab-treated subjects reported malignancies excluding nonmelanoma skin cancers. Nonmelanoma skin cancers were reported in 0.8% of treated patients. Again, patients must also be screened for latent TB prior to initiating treatment and antituberculosis treatment must be initiated for positive test results.

Ustekinumab is administered as a weight-based subcutaneous injection. For patients weighing ≤100 kg (220 lb), ustekinumab is given at 45 mg initially (week 0), 45 mg four weeks later (week 4), followed by 45 mg every 12 weeks for the duration of treatment. For patients weighing >100 kg (220 lb), ustekinumab is given at 90 mg initially (week 0), 90 mg four weeks later (week 4), followed by 90 mg every 12 weeks for the duration of treatment.

Selected Readings

Burmester GR, Mease P, Dijkmans et al: Adalimumab safety and mortality rates from global clinical trials of six immune-mediated inflammatory diseases. *Ann Rheum Dis* 2009;68:1863-1869.

Chaudhari U, Romano P, Mulcahy LD, et al: Efficacy and safety of infliximab monotherapy for plaque-type psoriasis: a randomised trial. *Lancet* 2001;357:1842-1847.

Ellis CN, Krueger GG, and the Alefacept Clinical Study Group: treatment of chronic plaque psoriasis by selective targeting of memory effector T lymphocytes. *N Engl J Med* 2001;345:248-255.

Gordon KB, Papp K, Hamilton T, et al: Efalizumab for patients with moderate to severe plaque psoriasis: a randomized controlled trial. *JAMA* 2003;290:3073-3080.

Gottlieb AB: Psoriasis. Immunopathology and immunomodulation. *Dermatol Clin* 2001;19:649-657.

Gottlieb AB, Hamilton T, Caro I, et al, and Efalizumab Study Group: Long-term continuous efalizumab therapy in patients with moderate to severe chronic plaque psoriasis: updated results from an ongoing trial. *J Am Acad Dermatol* 2006;54(4 suppl 1):S154-S163.

Gottlieb AB, Lowe NJ, Matheson RT, et al: Efficacy of etanercept in patients with psoriasis. Poster presented at American Academy of Dermatology, New Orleans, LA, Feb 22-27, 2002.

Intramuscular alefacept improves health-related quality of life in patients with chronic plaque psoriasis. *Dermatology* 2003;206:307-315.

Krueger GG: Clinical response to alefacept: results of a phase 3 study of intravenous administration of alefacept in patients with chronic plaque psoriasis. *J Eur Acad Dermatol Venereol* 2003;17:17-24.

Krueger GG, Ellis CN: Alefacept therapy produces remission for patients with chronic plaque psoriasis. *Br J Dermatol* 2003;148:784-788.

Krueger JG: The immunologic basis for the treatment of psoriasis with new biologic agents. *J Am Acad Dermatol* 2002;46:1-23.

Kupper TS: Immunologic targets in psoriasis. *N Engl J Med* 2003;349:1987-1990.

LaDuca JR, Gaspari AA: Targeting tumor necrosis factor alpha. *Dermatol Clin* 2001;19:617-635.

10

Lebwohl M, Christophers E, Langley R, et al: An international, randomized, double-blind, placebo-controlled phase-3 trial of intramuscular alefacept in patients with chronic plaque psoriasis. *Arch Dermatol* 2003;139:719-727.

Lebwohl M, Tyring SK, Hamilton TK, et al: A novel targeted T-cell modulator, efalizumab, for plaque psoriasis. *N Engl J Med* 2003; 349:2004-2013.

Leonardi CL, Powers JL, Matheson RT, et al, and the Etanercept Psoriasis Study Group: Etanercept as monotherapy in patients with psoriasis. *N Engl J Med* 2003;349:2014-2022.

Mease PJ, Gladman DD, Ritchlin CT, et al: Adalimumab Effectiveness in Psoriatic Arthritis Trial Study Group. Adalimumab for the treatment of patients with moderately to severely active psoriatic arthritis: results of a double-blind, randomized, placebo-controlled trial. *Arthritis Rheum* 2005;52:3279-3289.

Mease PJ, Goeffe BS, Metz J, et al: Etanercept in the treatment of psoriatic arthritis and psoriasis: a randomized trial. *Lancet* 2000; 356:385-390.

Menter A, Gordon K, Carey W, et al: Efficacy and safety observed during 24 weeks of efalizumab therapy in patients with moderate to severe plaque psoriasis. *Arch Dermatol* 2005;141:31-38.

Menter A, Gottlieb A, Feldman SR, et al: Guidelines of care for the management of psoriasis and psoriatic arthritis: Section 1. Overview of psoriasis and guidelines of care for the treatment of psoriasis with biologics. *J Am Acad Dermatol* 2008;58:826-850.

Menter A, Tyring SK, Gordon K, et al: Adalimumab therapy for moderate to severe psoriasis: a randomized, controlled phase III trial. *J Am Acad Dermatol* 2008;58:106-115.

Papp K, Bissonnette R, Krueger JG, et al: The treatment of moderate to severe psoriasis with a new anti-CD11a monoclonal antibody. *J Am Acad Dermatol* 2001;45:665-674.

Pariser DM: Management of moderate to severe plaque psoriasis with biologic therapy. *Managed Care* 2003;4:36-44.

Saurat JH, Stingl G, Dubertret L, et al, CHAMPION Study Investigators. Efficacy and safety results from the randomized controlled comparative study of adalimumab vs. methotrexate vs. placebo in patients with psoriasis (CHAMPION). *Br J Dermatol* 2008;158: 558-566.

Singri P, West DP, Gordon KB: Biologic therapy for psoriasis: the new therapeutic frontier. *Arch Dermatol* 2002;138:657-663.

Tutrone WD, Kagen MH, Barbagallo J, et al: Biologic therapy for psoriasis: a brief history, II. *Cutis* 2001;68:367-372.

10

Chapter 11

Scalp Psoriasis

P soriasis of the scalp affects at least 50% of all psoriasis patients (Figure 5-1, see color insert). It is often the initial presentation of psoriasis and tends to remain throughout the disease course. For many patients, the visibility of these lesions and their relative treatment-resistant nature make scalp psoriasis one of the more difficult aspects of their disease. Typically, scalp psoriasis is characterized as sharply demarcated erythematous plaques with white-silvery scales. It may also present as minor flaking and patchiness. The lesions often cross the hairline onto the face or behind the ears (ie, retroauricular). Pruritus may or may not be present.

Because of hair involvement, the vehicle of the agent is just as important as the active ingredient. The wrong vehicle can result in poor patient compliance and ultimately poor outcomes. Common vehicles include solutions, shampoos, foams, gels, lotions, oils, or sprays. Shampoos are often less effective in the treatment of scalp psoriasis because they are on the scalp for a short period, but they are useful as adjunct therapy. Ointments and creams are generally undesirable to treat the scalp because of their messiness when applied, except for some elderly patients with xerotic scalp who appreciate the lubricating effect of the thicker vehicle. Typical active ingredients include corticosteroids, keratolytics, coal tar, retinoids, antiyeast/antifungals, and vitamin D_3 analogues.

The treatment of scalp psoriasis consists primarily of topical agents (see Chapter 5). If the scalp psoriasis proves to be recalcitrant to the usual therapies, a suggested

Table 11-1: How to Treat Treatment-Resistant Scalp Psoriasis*

Step 1:

- Apply Taclonex Scalp® Topical Suspension once daily for up to 8 weeks, then switch to weekends only for maintenance.

  or

- Apply clobetasol (Clobex®, Olux®, Temovate®) (eg, foam, spray, lotion, solution) twice daily, up to 1 month, then switch to weekends twice daily.

- Optional: Apply calcipotriene solution twice a day, every weekday once clobetasol is switched to weekends only.

Step 2:

- Step 1 plus tazarotene gel (Tazorac®) once daily ('triple' therapy).

Step 3:

- Steps 1, 2 plus occlusion with shower cap.

Other Options:

- For thicker lesions with scale: Derma-Smoothe® oil, salicylic acid (Keralyt® gel, Salex® lotion), or lactic acid (do not apply with calcipotriene)

- 20% LCD in Neutraderm®

- Anthralin (Drithocreme®, Micanol®, Psoriatec™)

- Intralesional steroids

- Lesions recalcitrant to all topical regimens; systemic agent may be considered.

*See also Table 5-3. Treatment-resistant scalp psoriasis is defined as scalp psoriasis that is not adequately responsive to first-line therapy, eg, mid-to-high strength topical corticosteroids.

aggressive treatment for treatment-resistant scalp psoriasis (Table 11-1) is topical clobetasol, a super-high potency corticosteroid, either as solution (Temovate®), spray (Clobex®), foam (Olux®), or lotion (Clobex®). Topical clobetasol should be used every day, twice a day, up to 2-4 weeks at a time. It should then be replaced with a weaker topical steroid or be used on weekends only, twice a day (so that weekdays become a steroid holiday). This sequence assures adequate treatment time and reduces the concern for overexposure to corticosteroids. Pathologic adrenal suppression (as opposed to physiologic adrenal suppression) occurs when high or super-high potency corticosteroids are used for more than 1 month and used in areas >1% body surface area (BSA). This is usually not a concern if corticosteroids are used with the restrictions described (ie, 2-4 weeks use at a time). Skin atrophy of the scalp from topical agents alone is extremely rare.

Calcipotriene solution (Dovonex®) may be an option beyond the above regimen, ie, to the steroid holiday weekday part of the weekday/weekend regimen, and should be used twice daily. If this combination is still ineffective after 1 to 3 months, tazarotene gel (Tazorac®) can be considered once daily, provided that reproduction is not an issue (tazarotene is classified as pregnancy Category X). Additional options for improving scalp psoriasis therapy include occlusion with a shower cap, which is best done at night after applying the medication and left on overnight.

In May 2008, Taclonex Scalp® Topical Suspension, a new vitamin D analogue and corticosteroid combination product, was approved by the FDA for the topical treatment of moderate-to-severe psoriasis vulgaris of the scalp in adults ≥18 years. Taclonex Scalp® Topical Suspension is applied to affected areas of the scalp once daily for 2 weeks or until cleared. Available in bottles of 15 g, 30 g, 60 g, and 2 × 60 g, treatment with Taclonex Scalp® Topical Suspension may be continued for up to 8 weeks. The maximum weekly dose should not exceed 100 g.

Each gram of Taclonex Scalp® Topical Suspension contains 52.18 µg of calcipotriene hydrate (equivalent to 50 µg of calcipotriene) and 0.643 mg of betamethasone dipropionate (equivalent to 0.5 mg of betamethasone). Prior to using the product, patients should shake the bottle.

In a phase II study, patients (n=218) with scalp psoriasis were randomized to treatment with calcipotriene hydrate/betamethasone dipropionate (n=108) or betamethasone dipropionate alone (n=110). The treatments were applied once daily on the scalp for up to 8 weeks. The calcipotriene hydrate/betamethasone dipropionate scalp formulation showed a significantly higher efficacy than betamethasone dipropionate alone after 2 weeks (P=0.005) and at the end of treatment (P=0.042). The study concluded that the calcipotriene hydrate/betamethasone dipropionate scalp formulation was superior to betamethasone dipropionate alone when used once daily for up to 8 weeks in the treatment of scalp psoriasis.

Lesions with thick scale are problematic because the active ingredients in a topical agent may not penetrate thick scale adequately. In these lesions, the addition of a keratolytic, ie, 6% salicylic acid (ie, Keralyt® gel, Salex® lotion) can be used. As discussed in Chapter 5, do not use salicylic acid simultaneously with calcipotriene. A suggested schedule is to use a keratolytic in the morning and calcipotriene at night (see Table 5-3).

Suggested Readings

Buckley C, Hoffmann V, Shapiro J, et al: Calcipotriol plus betamethasone dipropionate scalp formulation is effective and well tolerated in the treatment of scalp psoriasis: a phase II study. *Dermatology* 2008;217:107-113.

Duffin KC, Krueger GG: Topical agents in the treatment of moderate to severe psoriasis. In: Koo JYM, Lee CS, Lebwohl MG, et al, eds. *Moderate to Severe Psoriasis*. New York, Informa Healthcare USA, 2009, pp 49-74.

Papp K, Berth-Jones J, Kragballe K, et al: Scalp psoriasis: a review of current topical treatment options. *J Eur Acad Dermatol Venereol* 2007;21:1151-1160.

Chapter 12

Nail Psoriasis

Nail changes are a common component of psoriasis and can be distressing for patients. For many patients, this is the only manifestation of their disease, making nail examinations and recognition of disease characteristics important aspects of clinical visits. Nail changes observed in psoriasis include oil spots, pitting, salmon spots, onycholysis, and subungual hyperkeratosis. Occasionally, patients will lose the entire nail (Figure 12-1, see color insert). Oil spots are semitransparent yellow or brown discolorations of the nail plate that were named because it looks like oil has seeped under the edge of the nail. Pitting is a deformity in which tiny, irregularly sized, shallow, round indentations are randomly distributed on the surface of the nail plate. Salmon spots are salmon-pink areas representing psoriatic involvement of the nail bed. Lifting of the nail plate, or onycholysis, is common, and refers to the separation between the nail plate and nail bed manifested by a whitish extension from the distal or lateral edge of the nail toward the cuticles. It is lined by an erythematous border, marking the proximal edge. Onycholysis is often seen in conjunction with subungual hyperkeratosis.

Hyperkeratosis is also associated with fungal nail infections, which should be ruled out with cultures. One clinical difference is in the texture of the hyperkeratotic material. Hyperkeratosis of fungal infections is usually 'cheesier' and easily scraped off, while psoriatic hyperkeratosis is drier and more adherent.

Treatment of nail psoriasis is largely unsatisfying and counseling for these patients needs to be directed at setting appropriate expectations. Most treatments have either a high failure rate or unacceptable side effects. Nevertheless, some patients prefer to make an effort at amelioration and some do achieve success. Patient counseling should include a discussion that nail disease originates with an inflamed matrix, so any treatment that is successful will undoubtedly be slow because of the rate of nail growth. Patients should understand that the existing nail first must grow out before changes can be seen, which may take up to 1 year.

Possible agents for treating nail psoriasis include the topical therapies described in Chapter 5: calcipotriene (Dovonex®), and topical steroids, tazarotene (Tazorac®), or anthralin (Drithocreme®, Psoriatec™); however, anthralin can stain the nail brown and topical steroids may induce atrophy of the surrounding skin. Much of the patient's treatment needs to occur overnight because of daily handwashing and frequent use of the hands. Patients can use either latex or cotton gloves to occlude their fingertips at night.

Selected Reading

Lowe NJ, Moy RL: Therapy of nail psoriasis. In: Lowe NJ, ed: *Practical Psoriasis Therapy*, 2nd ed. St. Louis, MO, Mosby-Year Book, 1993, pp 233-237.

12

Chapter 13

Psoriatic Arthritis

P soriatic arthritis is more common than previously believed. Current surveys estimate that up to 40% of patients with psoriasis also suffer from joint disease. Among patients with moderate-to-severe psoriasis, up to 50% can present with significant arthralgias or formally diagnosed psoriatic arthritis. Although neither primary care physicians nor dermatologists are certified in rheumatology, recognizing symptoms and the presence of arthritis is within their capability. Often these providers serve as patients' only access to appropriate referral and joint care.

One critical difference between psoriasis and psoriatic arthritis is that psoriatic arthritis can lead to progressive and often irreversible bone and joint destruction, while psoriasis does not generate such permanent sequelae. To prevent this destructive process, it is critical for patients with early signs and symptoms of psoriatic arthritis to be identified and treated promptly, preferably with a safe agent known to alleviate symptoms and prevent progression of irreversible joint destruction. Ask patients about morning stiffness, 'gelling' after rest, joint pain, joint swelling, fluctuations of these symptoms that correspond with changes in their skin, and family history of psoriatic arthritis. Constitutional symptoms are unusual in psoriatic arthritis. Patients should be examined for joint swelling, tenderness, reduced range of motion, as well as nail involvement, which often correlates with distal interphalangeal (DIP) joint involvement.

Psoriatic arthritis is a seronegative, inflammatory joint disease that can affect one or more joints, with a predilection for feet and hands, particularly the DIP joints (Figure 13-1, see color insert). Most patients present with skin disease first, but some present with simultaneous onset, and even fewer with joint disease that precedes skin disease. The latter diagnosis is a retrospective one, but patients complaining of joint pain should nevertheless be thoroughly examined for any sign of skin involvement, particularly in classic areas such as the umbilicus, scalp, gluteal cleft, elbows, knees, and nails to confirm the diagnosis.

There are five classifications of psoriatic arthritis (Table 13-1). The details of each are not as important as being able to recognize symptoms, which may indicate the presence of this disease and warrant a rheumatology referral. This is particularly important for primary care physicians and dermatologists who have the opportunity of seeing patients early in their disease process and preventing irreversible bony changes. Appropriate disease identification also allows for the selection of treatment that may be helpful for both skin and joints simultaneously.

Etanercept (Enbrel®), adalimumab (Humira®), and infliximab (Remicade®) are FDA approved for the treatment of psoriatic arthritis, and are good choices for the treatment of both skin and joints. These agents are examples of a class of drugs called DMARDs, which are known to prevent or minimize the progressive bony destruction characteristic of psoriatic arthritis. Even though dermatologists and primary care physicians are not experts in rheumatology, it is perfectly acceptable to choose such systemic treatments rather than choosing a treatment that addresses only the skin (ie, topical medications, phototherapy). If possible, arthritis treatments that can complicate the management of psoriasis, such as systemic steroids, should be avoided. These are helpful tips in managing patients with psoriatic arthritis, but are not a replacement for individual management by a rheumatologist.

13

Table 13-1: Five Classifications of Psoriatic Arthritis

Type I   Asymmetric oligoarthritis

- Accounts for 70% of psoriatic arthritis
- Typically involves 2-3 small joints of fingers and toes
- Leads to 'sausage digits'
- Can involve bigger joints asymmetrically

Type II   Symmetric polyarthritis

- Clinically indistinguishable from RA
- Associated with low rheumatoid factor titers and elevated ESR
- Female preponderance

Type III   Classic psoriatic arthritis

- Involves DIP joints
- Associated with severe nail involvement
- Male preponderance

Type IV   Deforming polyarthritis

- Severe erosive disease
- Leads to arthritis multilans or 'pencil-in-cup' deformities, telescoping digits, and 'sausage digits'
- Involves DIP joints

Type V   Spondylitis/Sacroiliitis

- Involves sacroiliac and axial joints
- Male preponderance

DIP=distal interphalangeal; ESR=erythrocyte sedimentation rate; RA=rheumatoid arthritis

Selected Readings

Andrews BS, Lowe NJ: Therapy of psoriatic arthritis. In: Lowe NJ, ed: *Practical Psoriasis Therapy*, 2nd ed. St. Louis, MO, Mosby-Year Book, 1993, pp 239-256.

Gladman DD: Psoriatic arthritis. In: Weinstein GD, Gottlieb AB, eds: *Therapy of Moderate-to-Severe Psoriasis*, 2nd ed. New York, NY, Marcel Dekker, 2003, pp 219-237.

13

Chapter 14

Psoriasis in Pregnancy

Patients with psoriasis who become pregnant often experience significant improvement in their disease. One proposed etiology of this phenomenon is the bolus of natural hormones produced during pregnancy. This has also been used to explain the postpartum recurrence or rebound that women experience when their hormone levels suddenly plummet. However, women who experience continuation of their disease, or even exacerbation, during pregnancy require treatment.

For mild psoriasis, many patients prefer to use only nonmedicated emollients during pregnancy to reduce the risk of systemic absorption and fetal exposure to drugs, even those that are considered to be safe. An algorithm for patients requiring treatment is shown in Table 14-1.

For moderate-to-severe psoriasis, either ultraviolet B (UVB) phototherapy or bath-psoralen plus ultraviolet A (PUVA) (see Chapter 6) is acceptable, safe, effective treatment for psoriasis during pregnancy. UVB is usually suggested first because it is a simpler, less time-consuming treatment and does not involve the use of any chemical agents. Bath-PUVA is often reserved for more severe psoriasis because of the extensive time commitment required and low exposure to psoralen. Oral psoralens have not been shown to increase congenital malformations, although they may be associated with low birth weight. Although there is no convincing evidence that psoralen causes birth defects, the use of oral PUVA therapy is not recommended if pregnancy is an issue.

Table 14-1: Treatment Algorithm for Pregnant Patients

First Line:	Topical medications (vitamin D analogues [Dovonex®, Vectical®] and topical steroids are Category C)
Second Line:	UVB phototherapy
Third Line:	Goeckerman day care
Fourth Line:	Bath-PUVA
Fifth Line:	Biologics (Category B)
Sixth Line:	Cyclosporine (Category C)

PUVA=psoralen plus ultraviolet A; UVB=ultraviolet B

Goeckerman day care is an excellent option for its safety and efficacy, but is less attractive to many patients because of the inherent time commitments.

Cyclosporine (Gengraf®, Neoral®, Sandimmune®) can be used if necessary. Data collected from the national pregnancy registry of transplant patients who took the drug throughout their pregnancies show that there is no convincing evidence that the drug is teratogenic. Low birth weight and premature births were the only consistent findings in this group of patients. Therefore, the FDA classified cyclosporine as pregnancy Category C, meaning that there was no convincing data in humans that cyclosporine is teratogenic. Nursing mothers should not use cyclosporine because it is secreted in breast milk.

Finally, several of the newer biologic agents such as adalimumab (Humira®), alefacept (Amevive®), and etanercept (Enbrel®) are pregnancy Category B.

Table 14-2: Treatments That Are Contraindicated During Pregnancy

Oral Retinoids:	Category X	Acitretin (Soriatane®)
		Isotretinoin (Accutane®)
Topical Retinoids:	Category X	Tazarotene (Tazorac®)
Methotrexate:	Category X	Trexall™

The same guidelines should be used for women who do not use adequate birth control or who are planning to become pregnant.

Physicians need to be aware not only of appropriate treatment options during pregnancy, but also which drugs are contraindicated (Table 14-2). Oral retinoids such as acitretin (Soriatane®) and the topical retinoid tazarotene (Tazorac®) are Category X and absolutely contraindicated during pregnancy, in women of childbearing age who do not use adequate birth control, or in those who plan to become pregnant during and within 3 years of discontinuation in the case of acitretin. The half-life of acitretin, the only oral retinoid now approved for the treatment of psoriasis, is approximately 50 to 100 hours. However, ingestion of alcohol during therapy promotes transesterification of acitretin to etretinate, which has a half-life of 120 days, and can be detected in the serum up to 2 years after discontinuation of treatment.

The topical retinoid approved for psoriasis is tazarotene. It is pregnancy Category X in the United States. This is because of possible systemic absorption of the drug and fear of teratogenicity as seen with the use of oral retinoids.

As with oral retinoids, women should have a pregnancy test before starting treatment and use adequate birth control throughout treatment.

Methotrexate (Trexall™) is known and used as an abortifacient. It can be teratogenic at low doses and is strictly contraindicated during pregnancy. Women should not take this drug during pregnancy and should not become pregnant for at least 3 months after discontinuation. Because of reports of sperm abnormalities, the same recommendation is made for men regarding fathering a baby while they are taking methotrexate and for 3 months afterward.

14

Chapter 15

For the Nonspecialist: When to Refer

Treating psoriasis with topical agents in patients whose disease involves >10% of total body surface area is usually not feasible. To estimate involvement, use the size of the patient's palm plus his or her thumb, which is approximately 1% of his or her total body surface area. Generally, nondermatologists have little expertise with phototherapy or other systemic agents for the treatment of psoriasis. Therefore, while it is still important to prescribe topical medications, it is equally important to recognize that patients with >10% body surface area involvement should be referred to a dermatologist for more definitive treatments such as phototherapy, systemic therapy, or Goeckerman therapy (see Chapter 8).

In some cases, even when involvement is <10%, psoriasis may be resistant to maximal topical regimens, or the patient may find his or her disease particularly distressing. In these cases, referral is appropriate for more sophisticated modalities. Systemic therapy may be appropriate in mild treatment-resistant cases in which a patient's quality of life (QOL) is severely disturbed because of the disease. Even small, recalcitrant lesions in sensitive areas, such as the scalp, genitalia, gluteal cleft, or hands, can be physically or emotionally disabling.

If the patient has significant problems with arthralgias or arthritis, referral to either a dermatologist, rheumatologist, or both is appropriate. Certain systemic treatments can be beneficial for skin and joint disease.

The Koo-Menter Psoriasis Instrument (KMPI) as featured in Appendix D may be helpful for a nondermatologist to determine when referral is indicated.

Summary of Prebiologics Use

Drug Name	Dose
Acitretin (Soriatane®)	***Recommended starting dose:*** 25 mg qd ***Maintenance:*** 10-25 mg qd (lowest dose that is adequate)

ALT= Alanine aminotransferase, BUN=blood urea nitrogen, CBC=complete blood count, FDA=US Food and Drug Administration, LFT=liver function test

FDA: FDA recommended guidelines
Optional: Some dermatologists recommend

Laboratory Tests

FDA:

- Pregnancy test
- Lipids
- LFTs

Common practice:

- As mentioned plus CBC
- If possible, do not use in reproductive women

Optional:

- X-rays (to check for diffuse idiopathic skeletal hyperostasis [DISH] syndrome)

Frequency

- Pregnancy test once when considering therapy, again immediately before therapy, and then periodically through treatment
  (if at all possible, do not use in reproductive women).
- CBC, lipids, and LFTs at baseline, 2 wk, 4 wk, 8 wk then once q 3 months if stable

(continued on next page)

Drug Name	Dose
Cyclosporine (Gengraf®, Neoral®, Sandimmune®)	2.5-4 mg/kg/d divided into 2-3 doses ***FDA guidelines:*** Maximum duration of uninterrupted use is 1 year at a time
Methotrexate (Trexall™)	***Test dose:*** 2.5-5 mg once ***Induction dose:*** 15-30 mg/wk (usually taken as divided doses within 24 h) ***Maintenance dose:*** May be less than induction dose

ALT= alanine aminotransferase, BUN=blood urea nitrogen, CBC=complete blood count, FDA=US Food and Drug Administration, LFT=liver function test

FDA: FDA recommended guidelines
Optional: Some dermatologists recommend

Laboratory Tests

FDA:

- BUN and creatinine
- Blood pressure
- Magnesium
- Potassium
- Lipids
- Uric acid
- LFTs
- CBC

Frequency

Before starting: Blood pressure and creatinine twice at least a day apart. Also BUN, magnesium, potassium, lipids, uric acid, and LFTs

For follow-up: Blood pressure, BUN, creatinine, magnesium, potassium, lipids, uric acid, LFTs q 2 wk for the first 3 months and then q 4 wk thereafter

FDA:

- CBC
- LFTs
- BUN and creatinine
- Liver biopsy
- Chest radiograph

Common practice:

- As previously stated w/o chest radiograph
- Hepatitis panel

Optional:

- Pregnancy test

- CBC at baseline and then every month
- LFTs, BUN, and creatinine at baseline and then every 1-2 months
- Liver biopsy at (1) pre-therapy or shortly after initiation of therapy (2 to 4 months), (2) after 1.5 g cumulative dose, and (3) every 1-1.5 g thereafter

Appendix B

Summary of Biologics Use

Drug Name	Dose
Adalimumab (Humira®)	*Loading dose:* 80 mg SC (one-time dose) *Maintenance dose:* Starting the following week, 40 mg SC every other week
Alefacept (Amevive®)	15 mg IM every week for 12 wk, which is an FDA-defined course of therapy

ANA=antinuclear antibody, CBC=complete blood count, CMP=complete metabolic panel, FDA=US Food and Drug Administration, IM=intramuscular, IV=intravenous, LFT=liver function test, PPD=purified protein derivative, SC=subcutaneous
FDA: FDA recommended guidelines

Laboratory Tests	Frequency
FDA:	
• PPD	• At the onset of therapy and then periodically
Optional:	
• CBC screening	• Optional, as per clinical judgment
• CMP with LFT screen	
• ANA screen	
• Influenza vaccination	
FDA:	
• CD4 screening	• Every 2 wk
Optional:	
• CBC screening	• Optional, as per clinical judgment
• CMP with LFT screen	
• PPD	
• ANA screen	
• Influenza vaccination	

(continued on next page)

Drug Name	Dose
Etanercept (Enbrel®)	*Induction:* 50 mg SC twice weekly for the first 12 wk *Maintenance:* 50 mg SC weekly
Infliximab (Remicade®)	*IV infusion:* 3-5 mg/kg at baseline, week 2, week 6, and every 8 wk thereafter
Ustekinumab (Stelara®)	*Induction:* 45 mg (<100 kg) or 90 mg (>100 kg) on week 0 and week 4 *Maintenance:* Same dose every 12 wk thereafter

ANA=antinuclear antibody, CBC=complete blood count, CMP=complete metabolic panel, FDA=US Food and Drug Administration, IM=intramuscular, IV=intravenous, LFT=liver function test, PPD=purified protein derivative, SC=subcutaneous
FDA: FDA recommended guidelines

Laboratory Tests	Frequency
FDA:	
• PPD	• At the onset of therapy and then periodically
Optional:	
• CBC screening	• Optional, as per clinical judgment
• CMP with LFT screen	
• ANA screen	
• Influenza vaccination	

FDA:	
• PPD	• At the onset of therapy and then periodically
Optional:	
• CBC screening	• Optional, as per clinical judgment
• CMP with LFT screen	
• ANA screen	
• Influenza vaccination	

FDA:	
• PPD	• At the onset of therapy and then periodically
Optional:	
• CBC screening	• Optional, as per clinical judgment
• CMP with LFT screen	
• ANA screen	
• Influenza vaccination	

Appendix C

Summary of Phototherapy Use

Treatment or Drug Name	Dose
Oral methoxsalen* (Oxsoralen-Ultra®) for PUVA	Weight-based dosing (see weight scale at the end of this appendix)
Narrow-band UVB	Refer to standard phototherapy textbook for dosimetry.
Broad-band UVB	Refer to standard phototherapy textbook for dosimetry.

ANA=antinuclear antibody, FDA=US Food and Drug Administration, LFT=liver function test, MED=minimal erythema dosing, PUVA=psoralen/ultraviolet light A treatment, UVB=ultraviolet B

Laboratory Tests	Frequency
FDA:	
• Ophthalmologic examination	• Ophthalmologic examination once a year prior to beginning treatment and at regular intervals throughout treatment.
• Routine laboratory tests (not specified) Consider ANA, LFT	
• MED, skin typing	• Prior to beginning treatment to determine initial dose.
• Skin check for suspicious lesions	• 2- to 3-month intervals
• MED, skin typing	• Prior to beginning treatment to determine initial dose.
• Skin check for suspicious lesions	• 2- to 3-month intervals

*Also known as 8-MOP
FDA: FDA recommended guidelines

Methoxsalen Dosing for Oral PUVA
(FDA guideline is about 0.4 to 0.6 mg/kg)

Weight (kg)	Weight (lb)	Dose
<30	<60	10 mg
30-50	66-100	20 mg
51-65	112-143	30 mg
66-80	146-176	40 mg
81-90	179-198	50 mg
91-115	201-254	60 mg
>115	>254	70 mg

The Koo-Menter
Psoriasis Instrument

The Koo-Menter Psoriasis Instrument (KMPI) has been developed to assist physicians in making decisions about whether the psoriasis patient can be adequately treated with topical therapy alone or whether he or she may need phototherapy or a systemic agent in addition to topical therapy. The KMPI is an integrated tool to help physicians perform a comprehensive evaluation of psoriasis patients including physical severity, QOL impact, and arthritis issues, and document the need for a more aggressive treatment.

Ultimately, it is a clinical judgment as to how aggressively the patient needs to be treated, and this decision should be made after taking into account all of the above-mentioned factors.

Koo-Menter Psoriasis Instrument

Patient Self-Assessment: Name: _____ Date: _____

Part 1: Quality of Life - Please answer each of the following questions as they pertain to your psoriasis during the past month. (Circle one number per question)

	Not at All				Somewhat				Very Much	
1. How self-conscious do you feel with regard to your psoriasis?	0	1	2	3	4	5	6	7	8	9	10
2. How helpless do you feel with regard to your psoriasis?	0	1	2	3	4	5	6	7	8	9	10
3. How embarrassed do you feel with regard to your psoriasis?	0	1	2	3	4	5	6	7	8	9	10
4. How angry or frustrated do you feel with regard to your psoriasis?	0	1	2	3	4	5	6	7	8	9	10
5. To what extent does your psoriasis make your appearance unsightly?	0	1	2	3	4	5	6	7	8	9	10
6. How disfiguring is your psoriasis?										
7. How much does your psoriasis impact your overall emotional well-being?	0	1	2	3	4	5	6	7	8	9	10
8. Overall, to what extent does your psoriasis interfere with your capacity to enjoy life?	0	1	2	3	4	5	6	7	8	9	10

How much have each of the following been affected by your psoriasis during the past month?

(Circle one number per question)

	Not at All				Somewhat					Very Much
	0	1	2	3	4	5	6	7	8	9	10

9. Itching?   0 1 2 3 4 5 6 7 8 9 10

10. Physical irritation?   0 1 2 3 4 5 6 7 8 9 10

11. Physical pain or soreness?   0 1 2 3 4 5 6 7 8 9 10

12. Choice of clothing to conceal psoriasis?   0 1 2 3 4 5 6 7 8 9 10

Total Quality-of-Life Score (0 – 120) ☐
*(Medical staff to calculate)

12-item Psoriasis Quality-of-Life Questionaire (PQOL-12), Copyright 2002, 2003, Allergan, Inc.

Part 2:
A. Using the figures below, place an "X" on the parts of your body that currently have psoriasis.

Front   Back

Part 3:
A. Have you ever been diagnosed with psoriatic arthritis?
Yes ☐   No ☐

B. Do you have swollen, tender or stiff joints (eg, hands, feet, hips, back)?
Yes ☐   No ☐

If yes, how many joints are affected? (Check one box)
1 ☐   2 ☐   3 ☐   4 ☐   More than 4 ☐

If yes how, much have your joint symptoms affected your day-to-day activities?
Not at all ☐   A little ☐   A lot ☐   Very much ☐

Once completed, please return to medical staff

STOP

123

Koo-Menter Psoriasis Instrument

Physician Assessment Name: _____ Date: _____

Part 1: Total Quality-of-Life assessment score (from part 1 of previous page) ➡ ☐☐

Part 2: Area of Involvement: % BSA (body surface area)		Part 3: In terms of psoriasis severity, does the patient have:	Check Answer	
	Note: Patient's open hand (from wrist to tips of fingers) with fingers tucked together and thumb tucked to the side equals approximately 1% of body surface area		Yes	No
Head ☐ % Head up to 9% of total BSA		Plaque, erythrodermic, or pustular psoriasis with >10% BSA involvement?	Yes	No
Anterior Trunk ☐ % Anterior Trunk: up to 18%		Guttate psoriasis?	Yes	No
Posterior Trunk ☐ % Posterior Trunk: up to 18%		Localized (<10% BSA) psoriasis but resistant to optimized attempts at topical therapy or physically disabling (eg, palmarplantar psoriasis)?	Yes	No
Right Leg ☐ % Right Leg: up 18% (includes buttock)		Localized (<10% BSA) but serious subtype with possibility of progression (eg, pustular or pre-erythrodermic psoriasis)?	Yes	No
Left Leg ☐ % Left Leg: up 18% (includes buttock)		Clinical evidence of psoriatic joint disease as assessed by physician (eg, examine IP, MCP, and MT joints of hands, wrists, feet, and ankles, plus patient responses from Part 3 of patient self-assessment)?	Yes	No
Both Arms ☐ % Both Arms: up to 18%				
Genitalia ☐ % Genitalia: 1%		Substantial psychosocial or quality-of-life impact documented by patient Quality-of-Life self-assessment score of ≥50?	Yes	No
Total BSA ☐☐☐ %				

124

Part 4: Is phototherapy an option?

	Check Answer	
	Yes	No
Is a suitable phototherapy unit readily accessible to the patient?	Yes	No
Does the anatomical location or form of psoriasis (eg, scalp, inverse, erythrodermic) preclude phototherapy?	Yes	No
Does the patient have the dedication, time, stamina, or transportation for phototherapy?	Yes	No
Has phototherapy, as monotherapy, failed in the past?	Yes	No
Is phototherapy contraindicated (eg, photosensitive drugs, history of multiple skin cancers)?	Yes	No
In your clinical judgment, is phototherapy likely to yield substantial improvement to justify its use before systemic therapy?	Yes	No

Physician/Nurse comments: _____

_____

_____

If at least one of the shaded boxes in Part 3 and 4 above is checked, then the patient is a candidate for systemic therapy.

CONCLUSION: The patient is a candidate for systemic therapy	Yes	No

© 2003 JYM Koo and M. Alan Menter

From Menter A, Koo JM, Kowalski J: Optimizing psoriasis severity assessment: an interplay between clinical evaluation and patient-reported impairment. Presented at: 10th International Psoriasis Symposium. June 10-13. 2004: Toronto. Canada.

Index

NOTES

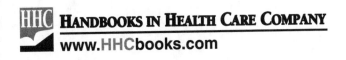
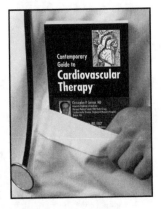

COLOR FIGURES

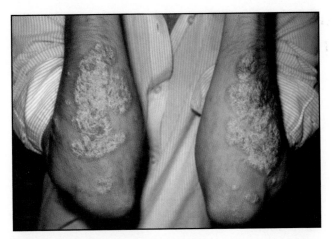

Figure 1-1: Plaque-type psoriasis.

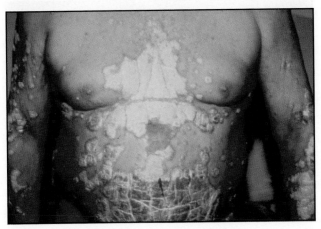

Figure 1-2: Severe, generalized psoriasis.

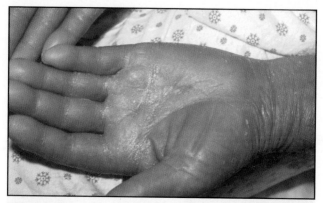

Figure 2-1: Carnauba wax appearance of pityriasis rubra pilaris.

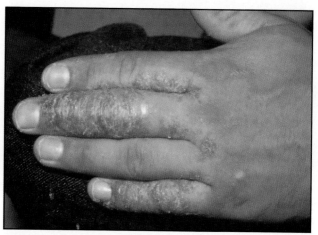

Figure 2-2: Hand eczema.

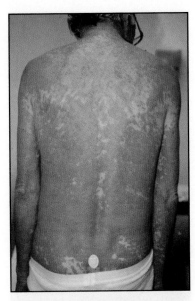

Figure 3-1:
Erythrodermic
psoriasis.

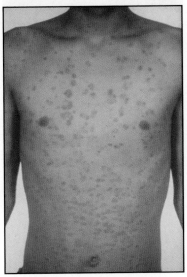

Figure 3-2:
Guttate psoriasis.

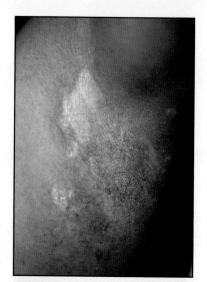

Figure 3-3:
Inverse psoriasis of the axilla.

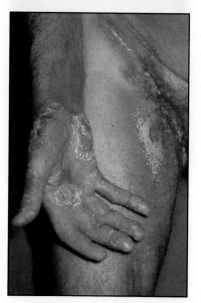

Figure 3-4:
Pustular psoriasis.

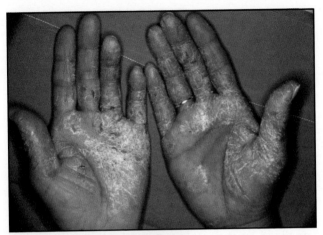

Figure 3-5: Hand psoriasis.

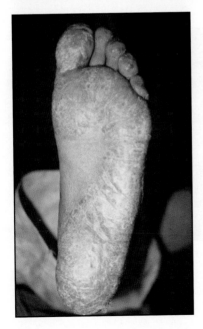

Figure 3-6:
Foot psoriasis.

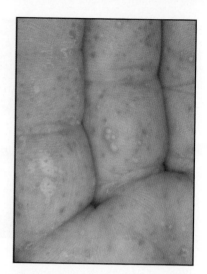

Figure 3-7:
Localized pustular hand psoriasis.

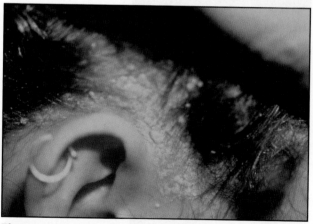

Figure 5-1: Scalp psoriasis.

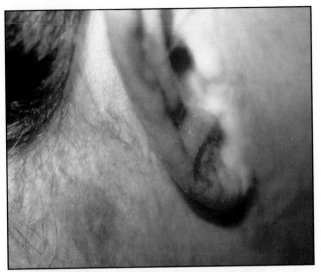

Figure 5-2: Skin atrophy (seen behind the ear) from chronic topical corticosteroid use.

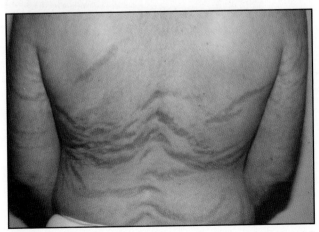

Figure 5-3: Striae from chronic topical corticosteroid use.

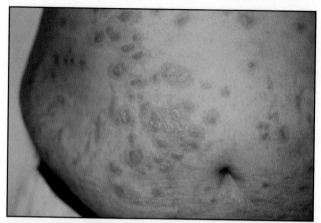

Figure 5-4: Perilesional irritation from calcipotriene.

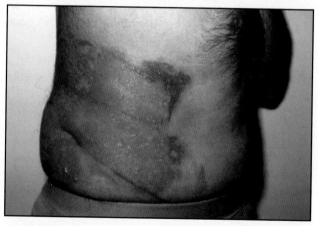

Figure 5-5: Perilesional irritation and pigmentation from anthralin.

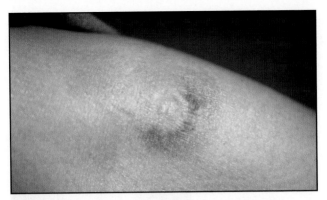

Figure 5-6: Perilesional irritation from anthralin.

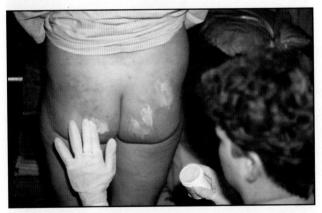

Figure 5-7: Application of anthralin.

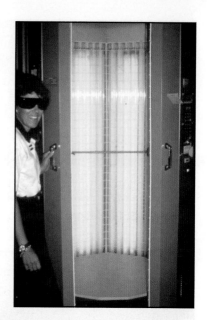

Figure 6-1:
Phototherapy unit.

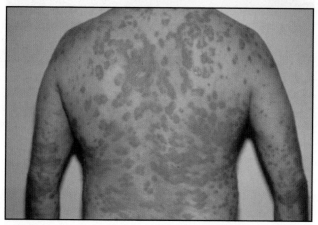

Figure 8-1: Generalized psoriasis before Goeckerman therapy.

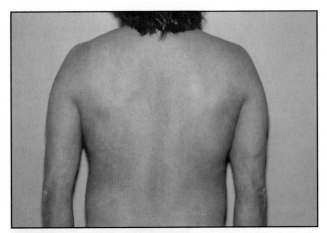

Figure 8-2: Generalized psoriasis after 28 days of Goeckerman therapy.

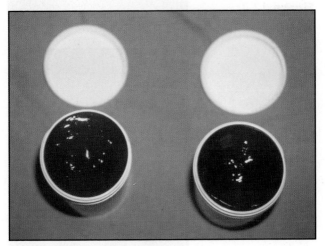

Figure 8-3: Crude coal tar.

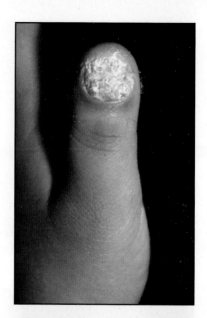

Figure 12-1:
Nail psoriasis.

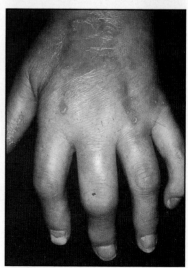

Figure 13-1:
Psoriatic arthritis with boutonniere deformity.